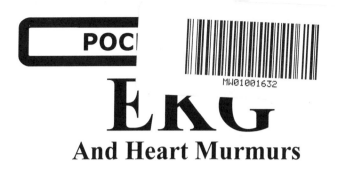

POC
EKG
And Heart Murmurs

Peter Q. Warinner, M.D.

WYSTERIA
Long Island, New York

www.wysteria.com

NOTICE:

Great care has been taken to insure that all of the information presented herein is accurate and up to date. Be aware that, with ongoing research, information is constantly revised, updated or otherwise changed. This publication is intended to be used as a guide by students in preparation for academic and clinical examinations. The author and the publisher disclaim any liability, loss, or damage incurred, directly or indirectly, due to the use of, or application of, this publication, or any of the information presented in this publication. This publication is not intended to be used as a treatment guide, for the management of patients, and therefore, should not be used as such.

Library of Congress Cataloging-in-Publication Data

Warinner, Peter Q.
    Pocket brain : EKG and heart murmurs / by Peter Warinner.
        p.   cm.
    Includes index.
    ISBN 0-9651162-3-9 (alk. paper)
    1. Heart murmurs--Diagnosis. 2. Electrocardiography. I. Title.
    [DNLM: 1. Electrocardiography--methods handbooks. 2. Heart
Diseases--diagnosis handbooks. 3. Heart Murmurs--diagnosis
handbooks.   WG 39W277p 1998]
RC685.V2W37   1998
616.1'207547--dc21
DNLM/DLC
for Library of Congress   98-31026
                                                                                    CIP

Printed in the U.S.A.
ISBN 0-9651162-3-9

CONTENTS

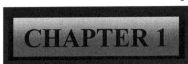

1

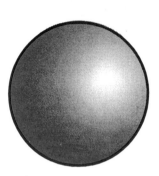

BASICS

BASICS

EKG or ECG = Electrocardiogram

I. <u>ELECTRICAL CONDUCTION PATHWAY</u>:

In a normal heart, depolarizations are perpetually generated in the Sino Atrial Node (SA Node). The rate at which these depolarizations occur is regulated by various factors such as nerves, receptors and chemicals that are beyond the scope of this text.

Depolarizations spread across the heart in a sequence determined by the anatomy of the heart's electrical conduction pathway. First, the atrial cardiac myocytes contract in unison; then the AV Node delays the deplarization until the atria finish contracting; then the ventricular cardiac myocytes contract in unison. After a refractory period, the cardiac myocytes repolarize in preparation for the next wave of depolarization.

1. **SA Node** (initiates depolarization)
   2. Right And Left Atrial Cardiac Myocytes
      3. **AV Node: "Junction"** (delays depolarization until atria contract)
         4. **Bundle of His**
            5. **Left Bundle and Right Bundle Branches**
               6. **Fascicles** (Right; Left Anterior; Left Posterior)
                  7. **Purkinje Fibers**
                     8. Right and Left Ventricular Cardiac Myocytes
                        (Endocardium first, Myocarium, then Epicardium).

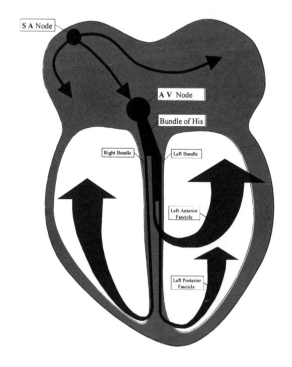

II. INTRODUCTION TO EKG LEADS:

Electrical activity moves through the heart, and subsequently through the body:
Each wave of depolarization that moves through the heart's electrical conduction pathway can be sensed as electrical activity in electrodes that are placed on the body. The quality and direction of this activity can reveal if the heart is normal or abnormal.

In order to get a three dimensional analysis, two groups of leads are used (see diagram):
1. The **limb leads** record activity in the coronal (frontal) plane of the body.
2. The **chest leads** record activity in the axial (horizontal) plane of the chest.

Leads are Bipolar configuration or Unipolar configuration (see diagram):
Bipolar configurations have one positive pole electrode and one negative pole electrode
    (Leads I, II, III, MCL1, MCL6 are bipolar).
Unipolar configurations have only one positive pole electrode because the center of the heart itself is used as a point of reference
    (Leads aVR, aVL, aVF, V1, V2, V3, V4, V5, V6 are unipolar).
Ground: In all configurations, there is a "ground" electrode used to establish a base line against background electrical activity (the right leg electrode is usually the ground).

Arrows are used in two ways:
    1. In the case of each lead, for illustration purposes, the arrow is always drawn to point to the positive pole, regardless of the direction of electrical activity going through the heart and body. This is illustrated on the next page.
    2. In the case of the heart itself, arrows are used as vectors to point in the direction of electrical activity. This can be positive (towards a positive pole) or negative (away from a positive pole) with respect to any lead. Ultimately, one arrow is used as a vector to indicate the direction of electrical activity as a summation of all leads together. This one, resultant vector is known as the **Axis**. The concept of Axis is described later.

Examples:

    Lead I
Electrical activity moving from right arm to left arm in Lead I (moving from the negative electrode of Lead I to the positive electrode of Lead I) is recorded as a positive deflection on the EKG tracing of Lead I. Conversely, activity moving from left to right is recorded as a negative deflection on the EKG tracing of Lead I.
    Lead aVF
Electrical activity moving downward through the body in Lead aVF (toward the positive electrode of aVF) is recorded as a positive deflection on the EKG tracing of Lead aVF. Conversely, activity moving upward through the body is recorded as a negative deflection on the EKG tracing of Lead aVF.

4

LIMB LEADS
Measure Coronal/Frontal Plane

Standard Leads: (Bipolar)
I (Left Arm Positive)
(right arm negative)
II (Left Leg Positive)
(right arm negative)
III (Left Leg Positive)
(left arm negative)

Augmented Voltage Leads: (Unipolar)
(Voltage is weak in these leads, so it is
augmented by the EKG machine)
aVR (Right Arm Positive)
aVL (Left Arm Positive)
aVF (Left Leg Positive)

CHEST LEADS
Measure Axial/Horizontal Plane

Modified Chest Leads: (Bipolar)
MCL1 (Right Sternum Positive)
(left arm negative)
MCL6 (Left Chest Wall Positive).
(left arm negative)

Precordial Leads: (Unipolar)
V1 (Right Ventricle)
V2 (Right Ventricle)
V3 (Intraventricular Septum)
V4 (Intraventricular Septum)
V5 (Left Ventricle)
V6 (Left Ventricle)

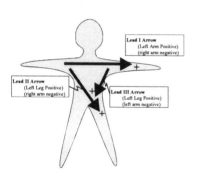

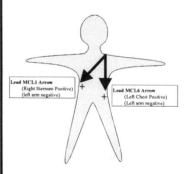

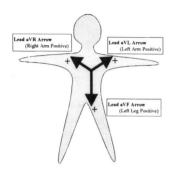

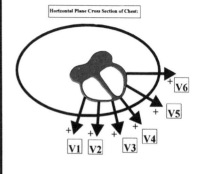

III. <u>EKG ELECTRODE PLACEMENT</u>:

<u>Reassure the patient</u>:
EKG machines record electrical activity; they do not send current through the electrodes.

<u>Prepare the patient</u>:
Clean and dry the skin at the sites where electrodes will be placed (alcohol is effective), shave hair if necessary. Electrodes may be suction cups that require gel, strap-on plates that require gel, or disposable tabs that adhere to skin. Protect the patient's privacy.

12 Lead Electrocardiogram:

Ten electrodes are placed on the body as shown below. The EKG machine uses various combinations of these electrodes to generate a graphic representation of 12 leads:

Leads I, II, III, aVR, aVL, aVF, V1, V2, V3, V4, V5, V6

Depending on the EKG machine, this graphic representation can be viewed on a monitor or printed out. Printouts are usually of two types: Some machines print out a continuous strip with each lead's graph in series; Other machines print out one page with all graphs arranged in a standard format, this format is shown in detail later.

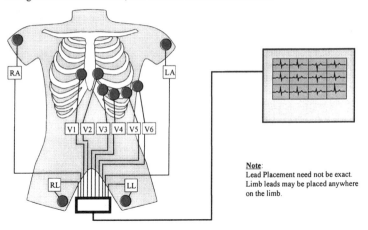

<u>Note</u>:
Lead Placement need not be exact. Limb leads may be placed anywhere on the limb.

3 Electrode Monitor:

Three electrodes are placed on the body as shown below. Depending on the electrode placement, the EKG monitor will generate a display of:

Lead II <u>or</u> Lead MCL1 <u>or</u> Lead MCL6.

Note that the graph of each lead can be seen on the monitor only one at a time. Usually, lead II or Lead MCL1 is used for continous monitoring situations.

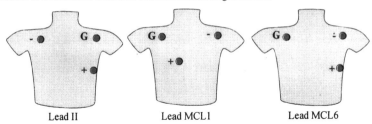

Lead II   Lead MCL1   Lead MCL6

IV. EKG GRAPH PAPER:

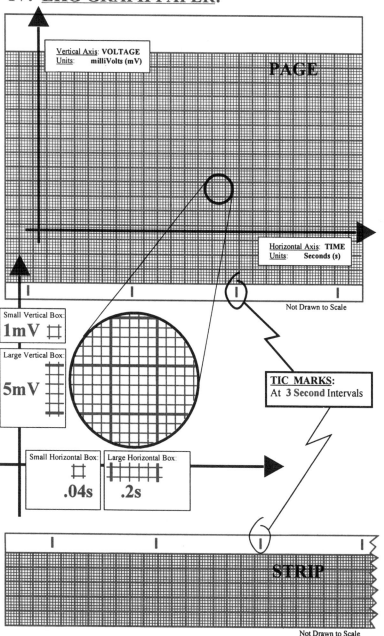

Vertical Axis: VOLTAGE
Units: milliVolts (mV)

PAGE

Horizontal Axis: TIME
Units: Seconds (s)

Not Drawn to Scale

Small Vertical Box:
1mV

Large Vertical Box:
5mV

TIC MARKS:
At 3 Second Intervals

Small Horizontal Box:
.04s

Large Horizontal Box:
.2s

STRIP

Not Drawn to Scale

V. THE 12 LEAD EKG GRAPH LAYOUT:

Since each lead records electrical activity from a unique point of view with respect to the heart, then the tracing that comes from one lead will look different from the tracing that comes from another lead. These differences allow for diagnostic interpretations.

Standard Layout:
In order to standardize the task of interpreting 12 lead EKGs, a standard layout has been adopted. The tracing for each lead will be located always in the same place on the page or strip as shown below. Each tracing is allowed to run for approximately 2.5 seconds so that at least one or two complete wave forms can be seen for each of the 12 leads.

Rhythm Strip:
This is a tracing obtained when any one lead (usually **Lead V1 or Lead II**) is allowed to run on much longer than the other leads (usually for 9 or 10 seconds). This is done to enable analysis of heart rate and heart rhythm.

12 Lead Page Layout:
There are four columns with three rows each: Leads I, II, III in the first column; Leads aVR, aVL, aVF in the second column; Leads V1, V2, V3 in the third column; Leads V4, V5, V6 in the fourth column. These tracings run for about 2.5 seconds each. A rhythm strip tracing runs for about 9 or 10 seconds across the bottom row.

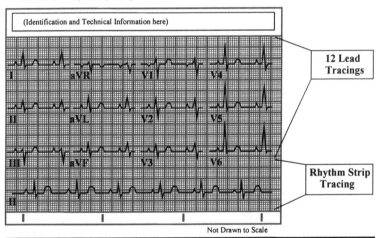

12 Lead Strip Layout:
This layout starts off with a rhythm strip tracing that runs for about 9 or 10 seconds. After the rhythm strip, tracings of the 12 leads run for approximately 2.5 seconds each. The tracings are in series according to the following sequence: Leads I, II, III, aVR, aVL, aVF, V1, V2, V3, V4, V5, V6.

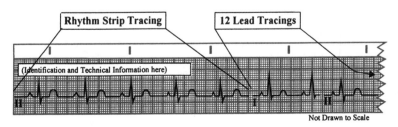

8

VI. NORMAL WAVE FORM:

For each heartbeat, as the wave of depolarization moves through the conduction pathway, the EKG leads record a characteristic pattern. This pattern is called the **wave form**. All wave forms recorded in the same lead will look exactly the same from heartbeat to heartbeat. However, as previously mentioned, any wave form recorded in one lead will look different from any wave form recorded in another lead.

A normal wave form is made up of several **component waves**. Each component wave corresponds to a specific event within the heart (as listed below). Each component wave is labeled with a letter (P, Q, R, S, T) in order to standardize diagnostic interpretations. The Q-wave, R-wave, and S-wave are considered collectively as the "**QRS complex**."

Component Waves:

-P-wave ....corresponds to **Atrial Contraction**.
-**PR Segment** between P-wave and QRS-complex corresponds to delay in the **AV Node**
-QRS complex ......corresponds to **Ventricular Contraction**
-**ST Segment** between QRS complex and T-wave corresponds to ventricular **Refractory Period**
-T-wave................corresponds to **Ventricular Repolarization**

(**Note:** An atrial repolarization wave is never seen because it is too small and gets obscured by the QRS complex).

Isoelectric Baseline: This is the line that is recorded when there is no electrical activity, it is seen on EKG recordings as the 'flat line' tracing seen between beats.

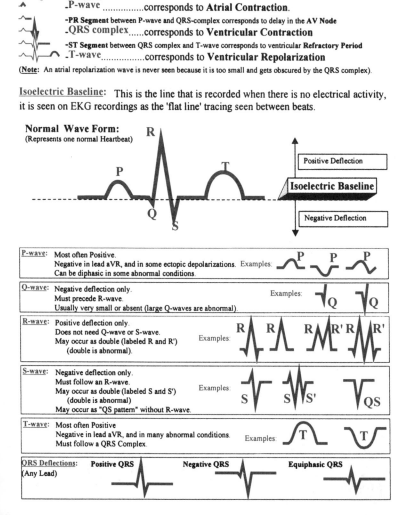

Normal Wave Form:
(Represents one normal Heartbeat)

P-wave:	Most often Positive. Negative in lead aVR, and in some ectopic depolarizations. Can be diphasic in some abnormal conditions.	Examples: P P P
Q-wave:	Negative deflection only. Must precede R-wave. Usually very small or absent (large Q-waves are abnormal).	Examples: Q Q
R-wave:	Positive deflection only. Does not need Q-wave or S-wave. May occur as double (labeled R and R') (double is abnormal).	Examples: R R R R' R R'
S-wave:	Negative deflection only. Must follow an R-wave. May occur as double (labeled S and S') (double is abnormal) May occur as "QS pattern" without R-wave.	Examples: S S S' QS
T-wave:	Most often Positive. Negative in lead aVR, and in many abnormal conditions. Must follow a QRS Complex.	Examples: T T
QRS Deflections: (Any Lead)	**Positive QRS** **Negative QRS** **Equiphasic QRS**	

VII. <u>INTERVALS AND SEGMENTS</u>:

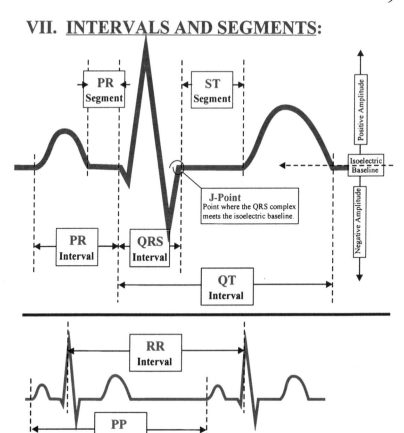

<u>Amplitude</u> = **unit of voltage** on the vertical axis.
   Positive Amplitude = height above isoelectric baseline (positive deflection).
   Negative Amplitude = depth below isoelectric baseline (negative deflection).

<u>Interval</u> = **unit of time** on the horizontal axis.
<u>Normal Intervals</u>:
   PR Interval: **<0.2** seconds (less than one large horizontal box): **aVR** is best.
   QRS Interval: **<.08** seconds (less than two small horizontal boxes): **V1** is best.
   QT Interval: **<0.4** seconds (less than two large horizontal boxes): **V1** is best.
   RR Interval: **0.6** to **1.0** seconds (between three and five large boxes): **II** or **V1** best.
   PP Interval: **0.6** to **1.0** seconds (between three and five large boxes): **II** or **V1** best.

<u>Segment</u> = any **portion of the wave form** delimited by specified points.
Elevations (positive deflections) or Depressions (negative deflections) are abnormal.
   PR Segment: isoelectric is normal.
   ST Segment: isoelectric is normal.

10

VIII. RATE:

One R-Wave signifies **One Heartbeat**.
Heart Rate Units = Beat Per Minute.

> ## Regular Rate =
> Heart Rate **60-100** beats per minute

> ## Bradycardia =
> Heart Rate **<60** beats per minute

> ## Tachycardia =
> Heart Rate **>100** beats per minute

METHODS OF RATE CALCULATION:

A. Counting RR Interval and Large Boxes:

Use the Rhythm Strip tracing, and locate an R-wave that begins near a Large Box line.
Count the number of Large Boxes that fit within the RR Interval (one large box = .2 seconds)
To avoid calculations, use the chart below to estimate the heart rate.

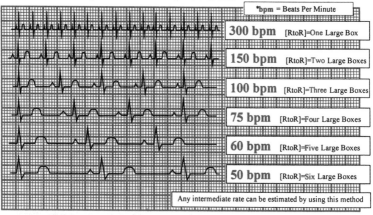

*bpm = Beats Per Minute

300 bpm [RtoR]=One Large Box

150 bpm [RtoR]=Two Large Boxes

100 bpm [RtoR]=Three Large Boxes

75 bpm [RtoR]=Four Large Boxes

60 bpm [RtoR]=Five Large Boxes

50 bpm [RtoR]=Six Large Boxes

Any intermediate rate can be estimated by using this method

B. Counting RR Intervals and Tic Marks:

Use the Rhythm Strip tracing, and locate an R-wave that begins near a Tic Mark (the 3 second interval marker).
Two Tic Marks = 6 seconds.
Count the number of RR Intervals that occur within 2 tic marks to obtain the number of beats in 6 seconds.
Multiply that number by 10 to obtain the number of beats in 60 seconds (Beats Per Minute).
This method is effective when the rhythm is irregular.

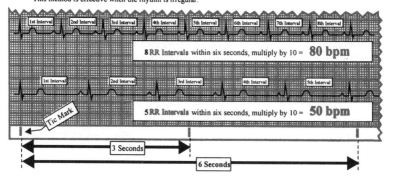

1st Interval 2nd Interval 3rd Interval 4th Interval 5th Interval 6th Interval 7th Interval 8th Interval

8 RR Intervals within six seconds, multiply by 10 = **80 bpm**

1st Interval 2nd Interval 3rd Interval 4th Interval 5th Interval

5 RR Intervals within six seconds, multiply by 10 = **50 bpm**

Tic Mark

3 Seconds

6 Seconds

IX. <u>RHYTHM</u>:

Rhythm:
The quality of timing as one heart beat is compared to the next, regardless of rate.
This is determined by comparing the length of several adjacent RR Intervals.
Described as Regular, Regularly Irregular, or Irregularly Irregular (as shown below).

Rate (as distinguished from rhythm):
The quantity of heart beats produced per unit time, regardless of rhythm.
This is measured by counting the number of R-waves per minute (beats per minute).
Described as Regular (60-100bpm), Bradycardic (<60bpm), or Tachycardic (>100bpm).

Regular Rhythm:
All RR Intervals of **equal** sizes within the same lead.
A rhythm strip tracing is used to analyze rhythm.

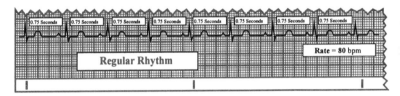

Regularly Irregular Rhythm:
RR Intervals of **different** sizes within the same lead, but there is **some overall pattern**.
A rhythm strip tracing is used to analyze rhythm.

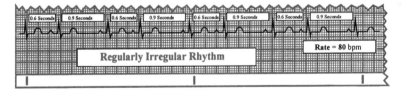

Irregularly Irregular Rhythm:
RR Intervals of **different** sizes within the same lead, and there is **no** overall **pattern**.
A rhythm strip tracing is used to analyze rhythm.

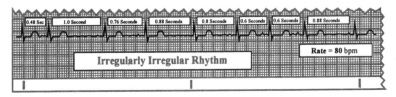

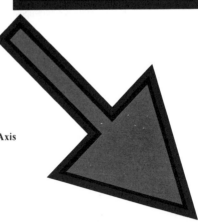

CHAPTER 2

QRS AXIS

QRS AXIS

I. Concept of Axis:

Axis: defined as the resultant vector obtained by the sum of all cardiac electrical activity. During one cycle, as the wave of depolarization activity moves through the electrical conduction pathway, the direction of this activity is constantly changing. However, the overall thrust of this activity, when added together, is in one direction. This is calculated and plotted as an arrow on the Axial Coordinate System. (Note: even though a vector is an arrow used to express magnitude and direction, it is the direction alone that is used for diagnostic interpretation of Axis.)

With each heartbeat, as each wave of depolarization moves throughout the conduction pathway, most of the electrical activity is directed towards the left ventricle. Obviously, the right atrium, left atrium, intraventricular septum and right ventricle all exhibit some depolarization activity, enough for contraction; however, the left ventricle exhibits most of the depolarization activity due to the thick myocardium required to eject and pump blood throughout the entire body.

For ease of understanding, the wave of depolarization is considered to branch out from the AV Node, like spokes from an axle. The depolarizations that go out to the right and left atria will have no effect because the atria are in their refractory period at that time. The depolarizations that go out to the right and left ventricles will cause ventricular contraction. Therefore, the ventricle which requires most of the depolarization activity is the ventricle which determines the direction of Axis. Since ventricular depolarization is recorded as the QRS complex on the EKG tracing, then the Axis is often referred to as the **QRS Axis Vector** or **Mean QRS Vector**. In a normal heart, since the left ventricle requires most of the depolarization activity, then the axis will point towards the left ventricle.

II. Axial Coordinate System:

The Axial Coordinated System is a two dimensional system of coordinates, similar to a polar coordinate system, used to graphically plot the QRS Axis Vector.

To create the system, a circle is superimposed upon the heart. The center of the circle is at the AV Node. The circle is made up of two 180° semicircles (the top semicircle as negative, the bottom semicircle as positive) for a total of 360° marked as shown below. Conventionally, the circle is marked at 30° intervals and divided into four quadrants as shown below.

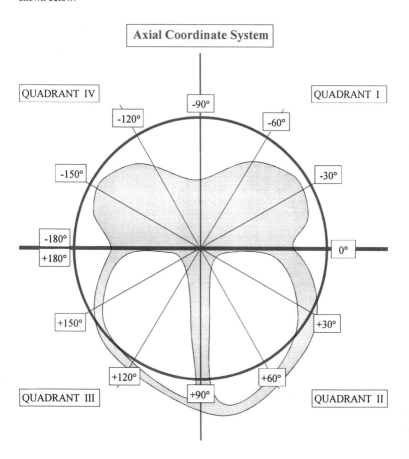

III. Calculating the QRS Axis Vector:

The QRS Axis Vector can be calculated using various methods and then plotted onto the Axial Coordinate System. The QRS Axis Vector is plotted as an arrow with the tail at the center of the circle, and with the arrowhead pointing outward like one spoke of a wheel. The direction in which the arrow points will define the QRS Axis in units of degree.

Clinical Correlation:

Every patient has a different QRS Axis. Furthermore, the QRS Axis that is calculated for one patient at one point in time may change for that same patient at another point in time. The value of the QRS Axis has diagnostic implications that are discussed later.

Note:

Displacement or malrotation of the heart causes inaccuracy of QRS Axis calculation. There are methods of correction, but it is beyond the scope of this text to present them.

IV. Lead I + Lead aVF method to calculate the QRS Axis:

Usually, the QRS Axis is analyzed in one plane only, the frontal plane. So, the frontal plane leads (limb leads) are used to calculate the QRS Axis. Each of the limb leads may be superimposed onto the circle that was previously described but, since the QRS Axis is calculated in a two dimensional plane, only two perpendicular axes are required. Therefore, **Limb Lead I** and **Limb Lead aVF** are chosen, and the Axial Coordinate System is modified as shown below.

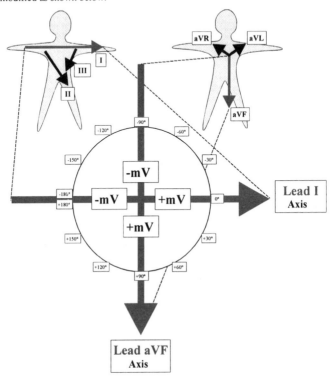

16

<u>Step by Step Formal Calculation</u>:
1. Look at the EKG tracing of **Lead I** to see if the QRS deflection is positive or negative
2. Count the net amplitude of the deflection in mV
3. Plot this as a vertical line on the Axial Coordinate System
   Note: **Positive** deflection in **Lead I** is plotted **right**ward on **Lead I axis**.
   If the QRS is **equiphasic** in **Lead I**, then plot a vertical line at **zero**.
4. Look at the EKG tracing of **Lead aVF** to see if QRS deflection is positive or negative
5. Count the net amplitude of the deflection in mV
6. Plot this as a horizontal line on the Axial Coordinate System
   Note: **Positive** deflection in **Lead aVF** is plotted **down**ward on **Lead aVF axis**.
   If the QRS is **equiphasic** in **Lead aVF**, then plot a horizontal line at **zero**.
7. A third line is drawn starting at the center of the circle and going through the
   intersection point formed by the first two lines.
8. This third line is the **QRS Axis Vector**. Extend this line until it crosses the circle.
9. The point at which it crosses the circle will be the degree of the vector
10. Note: if QRS is **equiphasic** in both I and aVF, then other methods must be used.

Examples:

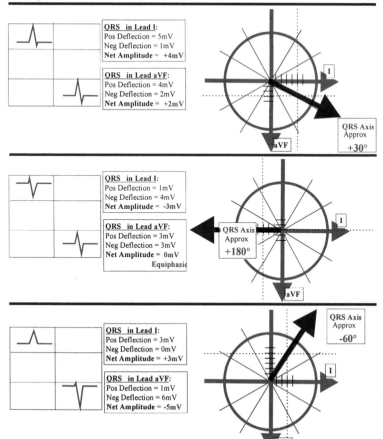

Step by Step Quick Estimation:

1. Look at the EKG tracing of **Lead I** to see if the QRS deflection is positive or negative
2. Look at the EKG tracing of **Lead aVF** to see if QRS deflection is positive or negative
3. Identify the quadrant that the QRS Axis Vector will lie in based upon the combination of positive and/or negative deflections of Lead I and Lead aVF as shown below.

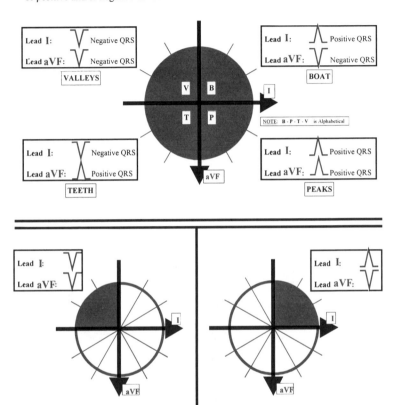

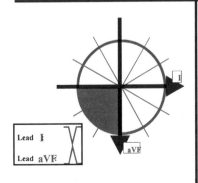

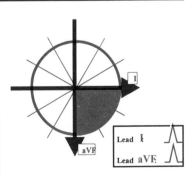

V. Alternative Methods of QRS Axis Calculation:

These three methods are based on a modified version of the Axial Coordinate System. In this version, all the limb leads are superimposed upon the circle which was previously described, so that the six limb leads become six axes. All the limb lead axes retain their orientation in the frontal plane, and retain direction in terms of positive/negative pole. Furthermore, the Axial Coordinate System retains its pattern of labeling in terms of positive/negative degree units.

This modified system, is sometimes called the **Hexaxial Coordinate System**, see the diagram below for more details.

This system can cause confusion. For example, when there is a positive amplitude in lead aVR or Lead aVL, this results in a negative degree of QRS Axis. See the following methods for further explanation.

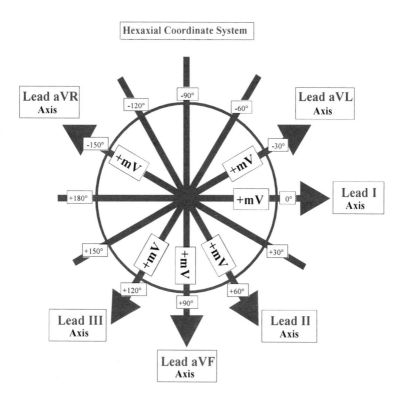

The Most Positive Method:

1. Among the six Limb Lead EKG tracings, identify the QRS complex with the most positive deflection.
2. Locate the arrow on the Hexaxial Coordinate System that corresponds to this Limb Lead.
3. The point at which this arrow crosses the circle will be the degree of the QRS Axis Vector.

Example:

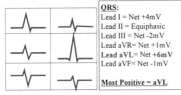

QRS:
Lead I = Net +4mV
Lead II = Equiphasic
Lead III = Net -2mV
Lead aVR= Net +1mV
Lead aVL= Net +6mV
Lead aVF= Net -1mV

Most Positive = aVL

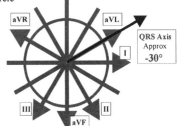

The Most Negative Method:

1. Among the six Limb Lead EKG tracings, identify the QRS complex with the most negative deflection.
2. Locate the arrow on the Hexaxial Coordinate System that corresponds to this Limb Lead.
3. The point at which this arrow crosses the circle in the **negative direction**, will be the degree of the QRS Axis Vector.

Example:

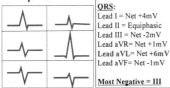

QRS:
Lead I = Net +4mV
Lead II = Equiphasic
Lead III = Net -2mV
Lead aVR= Net +1mV
Lead aVL= Net +6mV
Lead aVF= Net -1mV

Most Negative = III

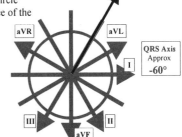

The Equiphasic Method:

1. Among the six Limb Lead EKG tracings, identify the QRS complex that is most equiphasic.
2. Locate the arrow on the Hexaxial Coordinate System that corresponds to this Limb Lead.
3. Locate the arrow which is perpendicular to this one.
4. Look at the tracing of the Lead that corresponds to this arrow to see if it is a positive or negative deflection.
5. If it is positive, then the point at which this arrow crosses the circle will be the degree of the QRS Axis Vector.
6. If it is negative, then the point at which this arrow crosses the circle, in the negative direction, will be the degree of the QRS Axis Vector.

Example:

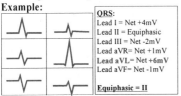

QRS:
Lead I = Net +4mV
Lead II = Equiphasic
Lead III = Net -2mV
Lead aVR= Net +1mV
Lead aVL= Net +6mV
Lead aVF= Net -1mV

Equiphasic = II

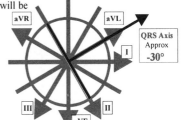

20

VI. Diagnostic interpretation of QRS Axis:

As previously mentioned, every patient has a different QRS Axis, and the axis that is calculated for one patient at one point in time may change for that same patient at another point in time. The value of the QRSaxis has diagnostic implications, there are normal ranges and abnormal ranges. **Normal QRS axis range** is 0° to +90°. This logically corresponds to the part of the circle that is superimposed upon the left ventricle.

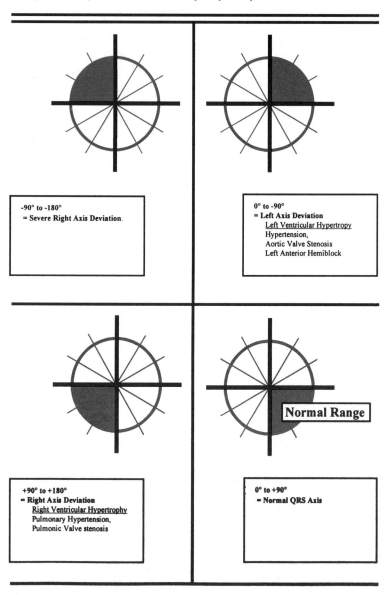

-90° to -180°
= Severe Right Axis Deviation.

0° to -90°
= **Left Axis Deviation**
 Left Ventricular Hypertropy
 Hypertension,
 Aortic Valve Stenosis
 Left Anterior Hemiblock

+90° to +180°
= **Right Axis Deviation**
 Right Ventricular Hypertrophy
 Pulmonary Hypertension,
 Pulmonic Valve stenosis

0° to +90°
= **Normal QRS Axis**

Normal Range

ENLARGEMENT

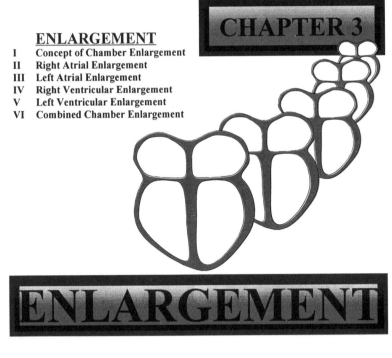

CHAPTER 3

ENLARGEMENT

I. Concept of Enlargement:

Cardiomyopathies of various etiologies may cause certain types of heart enlargement. More commonly however, there are pressure/volume overloading situations which cause enlargement of the heart chambers (right and left atria; right and left ventricles). This is then known as **"Chamber Enlargement,"** or just **"Enlargement."**

As the heart enlarges, the normal anatomy of the electrical conduction pathway becomes distorted. The EKG waveform shows characteristic changes related to the location of the distorted anatomy. Obstructive conditions that cause increased pressure within a chamber may be intrinsic to the heart (valve problems) or extrinsic to the heart (pulmonary or systemic hypertension). Beware: if the heart enlarges to the point where the coronary arteries cannot supply enough blood, then the heart is at risk for ischemia and infarct.

There are various terminologies used to describe these situations, but the anatomic changes and related EKG waveform changes are consistent. During atrial enlargement, the atria are said to dilate: the volume of the chamber expands under the force of chronic pressure overload, and the wall thickness becomes thin. During ventricular enlargement, the ventricles are said to hypertrophy: the volume of the chamber expands under the force of chronic pressure overload, and the wall thickness becomes more thick. Note, however, that the words enlargement, overload, hypertrophy and dilation are often used interchangeably even though there are subtle differences in meaning.

II. Right Atrial Enlargement: RAE
"Right Atrial Hypertrophy" RAH
"Right Atrial Overload" RAO
"P-Pulmonale"

Criteria:
1. **Limb Lead II:** (also Leads III, aVF)
   Tall P-wave
   Amplitude > 2.5mV.
2. **Pecordial Lead V1:**
   Diphasic P-wave:
   First part = tall **positive** amplitude.

Clinical:
- Pulmonary Hypertension.
      -(COPD)
      -Pulmonary Embolism
- Tricuspid valve stenosis
- Tricuspid valve regurgitation.

P-wave

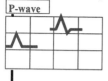

III. Left Atrial Enlargement: LAE
"Left Atrial Hypertrophy" LAH
"Left Atrial Overload" LAO
"P-Mitrale"

Criteria:
1. **Limb Lead II:** (also Lead I)
   Wide or Double Peak P-wave
   Interval > 0.11s
2. **Pecordial Lead V1:**
   Diphasic P-wave:
   Second part = **negative** amplitude.

Clinical:
- Mitral valve stenosis
- Mitral valve regurgitation.

P-wave

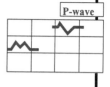

IV. Right Ventricular Enlargement:
Right Ventricle Hypertrophy RVH
Right Ventricle Overload
Right Ventricle Dilation

Criteria:
1. **Precordial Lead V1, V2:**
   Tall R-wave.
2. Precordial Lead V5, V6:
   Prominant S-wave.
3. Right Axis Deviation.

Clinical:
- Pulmonary Hypertension
- Pulmonic valve stenosis.

QRS Complex

V. Left Ventricular Enlargement:
Left Ventricle Hypertrophy LVH
Left Ventricle Overload
Left Ventricle Dilation

Criteria:
1. **Precordial Lead V5, V6:**
   Tall R-wave.
2. Precordial Lead V1, V2:
   Prominant S-wave.
3. Left Axis Deviation.

Clinical:
- Systemic Hypertension
- Aortic valve stenosis.

QRS Complex

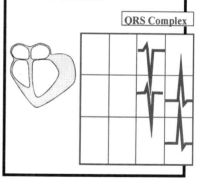

VI. Combined Chamber Enlargements:
Any combination of two or more of the above is possible:

        Dual chamber enlargement.

        Three chamber enlargement.

        Four chamber enlargement.

BLOCKS

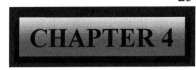

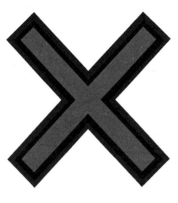

BLOCKS

I. Concept of Block:

The Electrical Conduction Pathway of the Heart may become damaged at any point along its route. This is then known as **"Conduction Block," "Heart Block,"** or just **"Block."** As a consequence, depolarizations become slowed or completely obstructed. When they become completely obstructed, an ectopic focus becomes responsible for depolarization:

An Ectopic Focus is any site within the heart (outside of the SA Node) that suddenly develops the ability to initiate depolarizations (atrial, junctional, or ventricular).

Atrial ectopic focus depolarizes at 60 bpm; but the rhythm is not normal sinus rhythm because the shape of the new ectopically generated p'-wave is different from the shape of the p-wave generated from the normal SA Node.

AV Nodal (junctional) ectopic focus depolarizes at 40-60 bpm, the rate is bradycardic, and the wave form shows normal QRS complexes but no p-wave, this is known as an "Idiojunctional" rate and rhythm.

Ventricular ectopic focus depolarizes at 20-40 bpm, the rate is bradycardic, and the wave form shows wide abnormal QRS complexes, but no p-wave, this is known as "Idioventricular" rate and rhythm.

NOTE: The atrial rate and ventricular rate may not be equal during blocks or arrhythmias
    Atrial Rate is determined by counting the number of p-waves per minute.
    Ventricular Rate determined by counting the number of QRS complexes per minute.

Often there is a correlation between the coronary artery blood supply and the electrical conduction pathway such that the cause of a specific conduction block can be traced to a blocked coronary artery, or to an area of myocardial ischemia/infarction.

Depending upon the location of the Block, the EKG recording will show characteristic patterns for diagnosis. These patterns are seen in the following rhythm strip tracings.

I. SINOATRIAL BLOCK (SA NODE BLOCK):

The term SA Node Block refers to a Conduction Block that occurs at the SA Node. It is the TP interval that is most effected by SA Block; in some cases the P-wave is absent. Either the SA Node does not generate a depolarization, or else the depolarization gets blocked from exiting the SA Node, but in either case the P-Wave is delayed or absent.

A. Transient Sinoatrial Block:

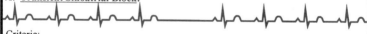

Criteria:
1. Absent PQRST waveform within an otherwise regular rhythm strip.
2. When rhythm is restored, the p-waves have the same shape as prior to the block.
3. When rhythm is restored, the rate is the same as prior to the block.

B. Sinus Block with Ectopic Escape Beats: (see arrhythmia chapter for explanation)

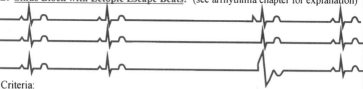

Criteria:
1. Absent PQRST waveform within an otherwise regular rhythm strip.
2. When rhythm is restored:
   The first **P-wave is different shape** from prior to the block (**Ectopic Atrial** Beat).
   Or, first no p-wave but a **Narrow QRS** complex instead (**Ectopic Junctional** Beat).
   Or, first no p-wave but a **Wide QRS** complex instead (**Ectopic Ventricular** Beat).
3. When rhythm is restored, the rate is the same as prior to the block.

D. Sinus Arrest with Ectopic Escape Rhythms: (see arrhythmia chapter)

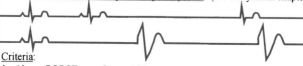

Criteria:
1. Absent PQRST waveform within an otherwise regular rhythm strip.
2. When rhythm is restored, a new rhythm begins:
   a. **Ectopic Junctional Focus:**
      Idiojunctional rhythm: no p-wave, narrow QRS complexes, rate 40-60bpm.
   b. **Ectopic Ventricular Focus:**
      Idioventricular rhythm: no p-wave, wide QRS complexes, rate 20-40bpm.

C. Sick Sinus Syndrome:

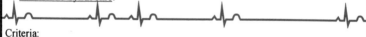

Criteria:
1. Variably absent PQRST waveforms due to a sporadically blocked SA Node.
2. The overall rhythm is **Irregularly Irregular**.
3. The overall rate is **Bradycardic**.
4. The ectopic foci are dysfunctional so there are **no escape beats or escape rhythms**.

II. ATRIAL-VENTRICULAR BLOCK (AV NODE BLOCK):

The term AV Node Block refers to a conduction Block that occurs at the AV Node. It is the PR interval that is most effected by AV Block. Depolarizations that come from the SA Node are delayed or completely blocked at or near the level of the AV Node.

A. First Degree AV Block: Known As: "1° AV Block"

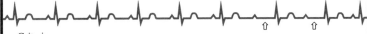

Criteria:
1. **PR Interval > .2s** (⇧)

B. Second Degree AV Block Type 1: Known As **Mobitz I** or **Wenckebach**

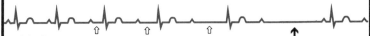

Criteria:
1. **PR Interval becomes increasingly long with each heart beat.** (⇧)
   (Therefore the PP Interval and RR Intervals become increasingly long).
2. The pattern culminates with an **absent QRS complex and absent T-wave.** (↑)
3. The PR Interval becomes normal again.
4. This overall pattern repeats.

C. Second Degree AV Block Type 2: Known As **Mobitz II**

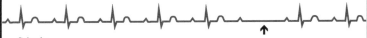

Criteria:
1. **PR Interval > .2s**
2. Atrial rhythm is regular (PP Intervals are equal from beat to beat).
3. **Random absence of QRS complex and T-wave.** (↑)

NOTE:
2:1 Mobitz II is a rhythm pattern with two P-waves for every one QRS complex.
3:1 Mobitz II is a rhythm pattern with three P-waves for every one QRS complex.

D. Third Degree AV Block: Known As **Complete Heart Block**

Criteria:
1. PP Intervals are equal.
2. RR Intervals are equal.
3. PR Interval is variable.
4. The P-waves and R-waves are "disconnected," they have no relationship.
5. Transmission of depolarizations is completely blocked at the AV Node;
   Therefore, an Ectopic Focus must initiate depolarizations which can spread throughout the ventricles in order to achieve ventricular contractions:
   a. Ectopic Junctional Focus: Narrow QRS complexes.
   b. Ectopic Ventricular Focus: Wide QRS complexes.
6. The Ventricular Rate is Bradycardic (superimposed on a normal atrial rate):
   a. Idiojunctional Rate (40-60bpm).
   b. Idioventricular Rate (20-40bpm).

III. BUNDLE BRANCH BLOCK (BBB):

This refers to a conduction Block that occurs at the Right or Left Bundle Branch. It is the QRS Complex that is most effected by a BBB.

A. Right Bundle Branch Block (RBBB):

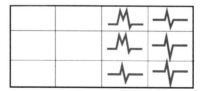

Criteria:
1. Wide, double-peaked R-waves in Precordial Leads V1 and V2: [QRS>.08s]
   (R-wave represents depolarization through Left Bundle).
   (R'-wave represents depolarization through Right Bundle).
2. Deep S-wave in V5 and V6.
3. Normal PR Interval.

B. Left Bundle Branch Block (LBBB):

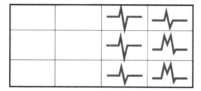

Criteria:
1. Wide, double-peaked R-waves in Precordial Leads V5 and V6: [QRS>.08s]
   (R-wave represents depolarization through Right Bundle).
   (R'-wave represents depolarization through Left Bundle).
2. Deep S-wave in V1 and V2.
3. Normal PR Interval.

IV. FASCICULAR BLOCK: Also Known as **HEMIBLOCK**
This refers to a conduction Block that occurs at the Level of the Fascicles.
The Left Anterior Fascicular block is most common.

A. Left Anterior Hemiblock:

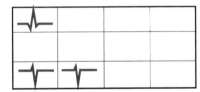

Criteria:
1. Left Axis Deviation.
2. Deep S-wave in Limb Leads III and aVF.
3. Sometimes Q-wave in Limb Leads I and aVL.

B. Left Posterior Hemiblock:
Criteria:
1. Right Axis Deviation.
2. Deep S-wave in Limb Leads I and aVL.
3. Sometimes Q-wave in Limb Leads III and aVF.

IV. COMBINED CONDUCTION BLOCK:
Any combination of SA Block, AV Block, or Fascicular Block is possible.

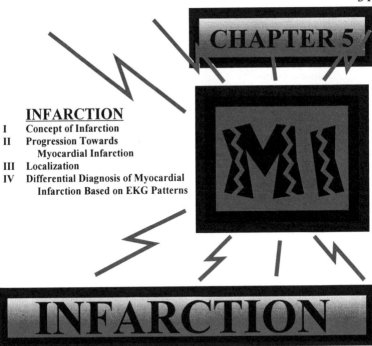

CHAPTER 5

INFARCTION
I   Concept of Infarction
II   Progression Towards
      Myocardial Infarction
III   Localization
IV   Differential Diagnosis of Myocardial
      Infarction Based on EKG Patterns

INFARCTION

I. Concept of Infarction:
"Heart Attack" is Myocardial Infarction (MI). Insufficient or blocked coronary arteries can cause injury to myocardium. If injury is prolonged, it progresses to ischemia and then to infarction. Infarction is irreversible death to an area of myocardium. Injured, ischemic, or infarcted myocardial cells cannot depolarize normally. The EKG waveform shows characteristic changes related to the progression towards and location of infarction. Localization is usually analyzed with respect to the left ventricle.

During coronary artery disease, blocked arteries cannot deliver blood to the myocardium. During some types of angina where the coronary arteries are stenotic or have spasms, the blood supply to the myocardium gets cut off abruptly. During chamber enlargement conditions and some cardiomyopathies, the coronary blood supply is insufficient to keep up with the expanded tissues. These and similar situations can lead to myocardial ischemia and infarction.

If the area of ischemia or infarction involves the electrical conduction pathway, then heart blocks or arrhythmias may result (however, ischemia/infarction is not a necessary cause of heart blocks and arrhythmis). If the area of infarction is extensive, then a ventricular aneurysm may result which can dilate and rupture.

Some Facts About **Significant Q-waves**:
1. Indicates acute MI when occurs with ST-segment elevation in the same lead.
2. Indicates old MI when ST-segment normal, or T-wave inverted in the same lead.
3. Defined as having **duration > 0.04 sec**.
4. Defined as having **depth > 1/4 of R-wave** amplitude in the same lead.
5. Never significant when it occurs in lead aVR.
6. In case of LBBB, Q-wave can be hidden by the right ventricular QRS complex.

II. Progression Towards Myocardial Infarction:

Two patterns of infarction are considered:
1. **Transmural Myocardial Infarction ("Q-wave Infarction"):**
   Damage to myocardial tissue extends through the full thickness of ventricle wall, from endocardium to epicardium.
2. **Subendocardial Myocardial Infarction ("Non Q-wave Infarction"):**
   Damage to myocardial tissue involves myocardium near the endocardium, and does not extend to the epicardium.

Damage progresses in four discrete stages:
1. **Ischemia** (reversible hypoxia from decreased blood flow)
2. **Injury** (reversible anoxia)
3. **Acute Infarction** (Irreversible Necrosis)
4. **Old Infarction Scar** (Irreversible Fibrosis; may cause Aneurysm)

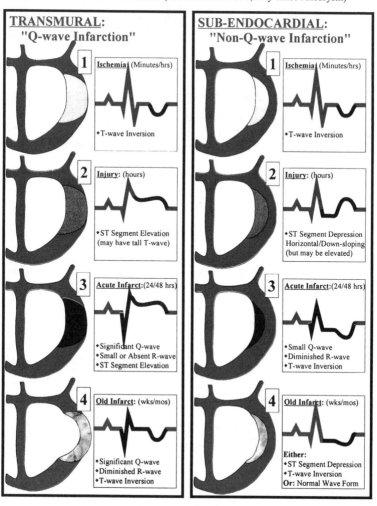

TRANSMURAL:
"Q-wave Infarction"

1 Ischemia (Minutes/hrs)
- T-wave Inversion

2 Injury: (hours)
- ST Segment Elevation (may have tall T-wave)

3 Acute Infarct: (24/48 hrs)
- Significant Q-wave
- Small or Absent R-wave
- ST Segment Elevation

4 Old Infarct: (wks/mos)
- Significant Q-wave
- Diminished R-wave
- T-wave Inversion

SUB-ENDOCARDIAL:
"Non-Q-wave Infarction"

1 Ischemia (Minutes/hrs)
- T-wave Inversion

2 Injury: (hours)
- ST Segment Depression Horizontal/Down-sloping (but may be elevated)

3 Acute Infarct: (24/48 hrs)
- Small Q-wave
- Diminished R-wave
- T-wave Inversion

4 Old Infarct: (wks/mos)
Either:
- ST Segment Depression
- T-wave Inversion
Or: Normal Wave Form

III. <u>Localization</u>:

The characteristic progression of EKG wave forms corresponding to myocardial tissue damage (transmural or sub-endocardial) is recorded in EKG tracings by the overlying electrodes. The leads that incorporate these electrodes show the characteristic patterns. The other leads show reciprocal reactions (tall T-waves, tall R-waves, ST depressions). These reciprocal reactions are variable and their analysis is beyond the scope of this text.

Furthermore, once the anatomic location of myocardial tissue damage is identified, then the coronary artery which supplies that area of ventricle is recognized as being occluded. **The charts below show which leads relate to which location and to which artery:**

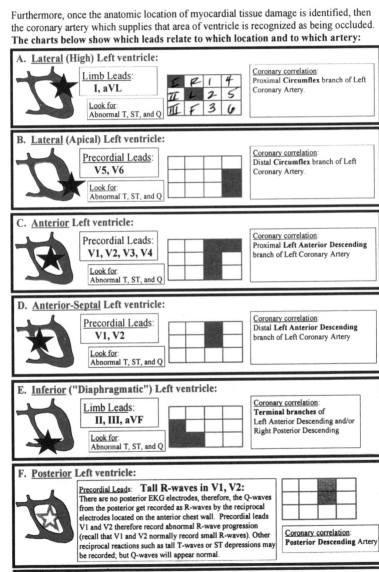

A. <u>Lateral</u> (High) Left ventricle:

Limb Leads:
I, aVL

Look for:
Abnormal T, ST, and Q

Coronary correlation:
Proximal **Circumflex** branch of Left Coronary Artery.

B. <u>Lateral</u> (Apical) Left ventricle:

Precordial Leads:
V5, V6

Look for:
Abnormal T, ST, and Q

Coronary correlation:
Distal **Circumflex** branch of Left Coronary Artery.

C. <u>Anterior</u> Left ventricle:

Precordial Leads:
V1, V2, V3, V4

Look for:
Abnormal T, ST, and Q

Coronary correlation:
Proximal **Left Anterior Descending** branch of Left Coronary Artery

D. <u>Anterior-Septal</u> Left ventricle:

Precordial Leads:
V1, V2

Look for:
Abnormal T, ST, and Q

Coronary correlation:
Distal **Left Anterior Descending** branch of Left Coronary Artery

E. <u>Inferior</u> ("Diaphragmatic") Left ventricle:

Limb Leads:
II, III, aVF

Look for:
Abnormal T, ST, and Q

Coronary correlation:
Terminal branches of Left Anterior Descending and/or Right Posterior Descending

F. <u>Posterior</u> Left ventricle:

Precordial Leads: **Tall R-waves in V1, V2:**
There are no posterior EKG electrodes, therefore, the Q-waves from the posterior get recorded as R-waves by the reciprocal electrodes located on the anterior chest wall. Precordial leads V1 and V2 therefore record abnormal R-wave progression (recall that V1 and V2 normally record small R-waves). Other reciprocal reactions such as tall T-waves or ST depressions may be recorded; but Q-waves will appear normal.

Coronary correlation:
Posterior Descending Artery

G. <u>Combination</u>: Any possible combination of the above is possible for multiple sites of tissue damage; for old and new infarcts together, and for multiple sites of occlusion

IV. Differential Diagnosis of Myocardial Infarction Based on EKG Patterns:

A. Pericarditis:

Acute:

<u>Wave Form</u>: Characteristic concave ST Segment Elevations.

<u>Localization</u>: Recorded in almost all leads (non-localizing).

<u>Other Findings</u>:
- ◆Auscultation of Pericardial Friction Rub.
- ◆Long periods of Pleuritic Chest Pain.
- ◆Normal Coronary Arteries, No Infarction.

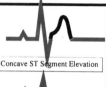

Concave ST Segment Elevation

Chronic:

<u>Wave Form</u>: T-wave Inversion.

<u>Localization</u>: Recorded in almost all leads (non-localizing).

Eventual T-wave Inversion

B. IHSS (Idiopathic Hypertrophic Subaortic Stenosis):

<u>Wave Form</u>: Significant Q-waves.

<u>Localization</u>: Recorded in Limb Leads II, III, aVF
and most Precordial Leads V1-V6.

<u>Other Findings</u>:
- ◆Harsh Systolic Murmur at Left Sternal Border.
- ◆Massive Septal Hypertrophy.
- ◆Normal Coronary Arteries, No Infarction.

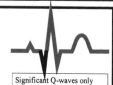

Significant Q-waves only

C. Chronic Stable Angina Pectoris:

<u>Wave Form at Rest</u>: Normal EKG.

<u>Wave Form at Stress</u>: Horizontal or Down sloping ST Segment Depression,
and sometimes T-wave Inversion.

<u>Localization</u>: Recorded in Leads corresponding to **coronary artery stenosis**.

<u>Other Findings</u>:
- ◆Physiologically, Emotionally, or Chemically Induced Chest "Pressure."
- ◆Episodic symptoms have duration of 1-5 minutes and are relieved by rest.
- ◆Coronary Stenosis, Myocardial Ischemia, No Infarction.

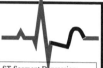

ST Segment Depression:
>1mV @ 0.08 sec after QRS

D. Variant "Prinzmetal's" Angina:

<u>Wave Form with no symptoms</u>: Normal EKG.

<u>Wave Form with symptoms</u>: ST Segment Elevation; sometimes T-wave Inversion.

<u>Localization</u>: Recorded in Leads corresponding to **coronary artery spasm**.

<u>Other Findings</u>:
- ◆Chest "Pressure" occurs at random during rest or during stress.

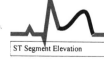

ST Segment Elevation

- ◆Episodic symptoms have duration of 1-5 minutes, and may be accompanied by shortness of breath.
- ◆Coronary Artery Spasm, Coronary Stenosis, Myocardial Ischemia, No Infarction, but infarction is possible.

E. Unstable Angina Pectoris:

<u>Wave Form at Rest</u>: Normal or Abnormal ST Segments and T-waves.

<u>Wave Form at Stress</u>: ST Segment Elevation and/or T-wave Inversions.

<u>Localization</u>: Recorded in Leads corresponding to severe coronary artery stenosis.

<u>Other Findings</u>:

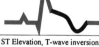

ST Elevation, T-wave inversion

- ◆Chest "Pressure" occurs during mild stress, and sometimes at rest.
- ◆May have history of Stable Angina that has progressed to more frequent symptoms; or may be new rapid onset.
- ◆Severe Coronary Stenosis, Myocardial Ischemia, History of past Infarction or may be pending new infarction.

B. Miscellaneous Summaries:

T-wave Inversions:	ST Segment Elevations:	ST Segment Depressions:
Myocardial Ischemia	Myocardial Injury	Myocardial Ischemia
Non-Q-wave Infarct	Q-wave Infarct	Non-Q-wave injury/infarct
Chronic Pericarditis	Acute Pericarditis	Stable Angina
Variant and Unstable Angina	Variant and Unstable Angina	Ventricular Hypertrophy
Ventricular Hypertrophy	Ventricular Aneurysm	Bundle Branch Blocks
Bundle Branch Blocks	Normal Variant:	Digitalis
Sub-Arachnoid Hemorrhage	Early Repolarization	
Pulmonary Embolism	in Leads V2,V3,V4.	Significant Q-waves:
Normally Inverted in Lead aVR		Q-wave Infarct
Normal Variant:		IHSS
in Leads III, aVL, aVF, V1, V2.		Pulmonary Embolism Lead III
Many other conditions		Normal Variant in Lead aVR
		Insignificant if seen in LBBB

CHAPTER 6

ARRHYTHMIAS

I   Concept of Arrhythmia
II   Arrhythmias Organized by Location
VI   Arryhthmias Organized by Rate

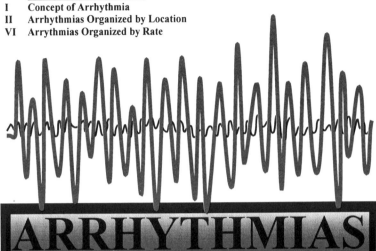

ARRHYTHMIAS

I. Concept of Arrhythmia: **"A Heart Divided Against Itself Cannot Beat"**
For each normal heartbeat, cardiac myocytes work together in sequence to eject blood.
Each wave of depolarization initiated by the SA Node gets sequentially delivered through
the anatomy of the electrical conduction pathway to each cardiac myocyte. But, if the SA
Node gets competition from ectopic foci, or if the sequence of depolarization is disrupted
or circumnavigated, then blocks and/or arrhythmias occur.

TERMINOLOGY: (as related to cardiac arrhythmias):
    Rhythm: the shape of the PQRST wave form, and how it changes from beat to beat.
    Normal Sinus Rhythm: the normal shape of the PQRST wave form, at a regular rate.
        (In Normal Sinus Rhythm, depolarizations eminate only from the SA Node).
    Arrhythmia: absence of normal rhythm (abnormal shape of the PQRST wave form).
    Dysrrhythmia: abnormal rhythm (used synonymously with arrhythmia).
    Asystole: absence of rhythm ("Flat Line").
    Ectopic Focus: (also called "Automaticity" or "Ectopy")
        Depolarizations initiated outside of the SA Node are called ectopic.
        ▪**Atrial Ectopic Focus:** shape of the **P'-wave** is different from SA Node P-wave.
            (Ectopics from inferior left atrium will cause an inverted P'-wave.)
        ▪**AV Nodal Ectopic Focus** has a **Narrow QRS complex** (normal), and no P-wave.
        ▪**Ventricular Ectopic Focus** has a **Wide QRS complex**, and no P-wave.
    Paroxysmal: change of rhythm with sudden onset, but not sustained.
    Escape Beat: If there is a block, some ectopic focus may initiate depolarization.
    Premature Contraction: Ectopic focus initiates depolarization before SA Node does.
        Atrial Ectopic (PAC), Junctional Ectopic (PJC), Ventricular Ectopic (PVC).
    Reentry: A depolarization that is delayed in a zone of abnormal conduction, as the
       rest of the heart deplarizes, may exit that zone and reenter normal tissue to cause a
       premature contraction. Reentry may also occur via accesory conduction pathways.

36

II. ARRHYTHMIAS ORGANIZED BY LOCATION:
A. Atrial Depolarizations going to the AV Node:

---

1. Normal Sinus Rhythm:

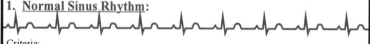

Criteria:
1. Rate above 60 bpm, and below 100 bpm.
2. There is a QRS complex after every P-wave, and P-wave before every QRS complex.
3. All P-waves are of identical shape because all depolarizations come from SA Node.
4. All RR intervals are equal.
5. All other intervals and segments are within normal ranges.

---

2. Sinus Bradycardia:

Criteria:
1. **Rate below 60 bpm.**
2. There is a QRS complex after every P-wave, and P-wave before every QRS complex.
3. All P-waves are of identical shape.
4. All RR intervals are equal.
5. All other intervals and segments are within normal ranges.

---

3. Sinus Block with Ectopic Atrial Escape Beat: (see Conduction Block chapter)

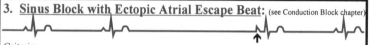

Criteria:
1. There is an abnormal pause after the T-wave due to lack of an SA Nodal P-wave, this causes a temporary lengthening of the RR Interval.
2. Since the SA Node refuses to initiate depolarization, the pause is broken by a new depolarization which is initiated by an ectopic atrial focus:
NOTE: **The ectopic P'-wave shape is different from the SA-Nodal P-wave shape.**
NOTE: Contrast this with **Sick Sinus Syndrome** where a dysfunctional SA-Node causes a repetitive partial Sinus Block in the absence of any ectopic escape beats. This results in an Irregularly Irregular Sinus Bradycardia Arrhythmia.

---

4. Sinus Arrhythmia: ("Physiologic Arrhythmia")

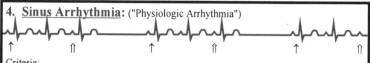

Criteria:
1. **Regularly Irregular Rhythm.**
2. The rhythm varies according to the pattern of **Inhalation (↑)** and **Exhalation (⇑)**.

---

5. Sinus Tachycardia:

Criteria:
1. **Rate above 100 bpm.**
2. There is a QRS complex after every P-wave, and P-wave before every QRS complex.
3. All P-waves are of identical shape.
4. All RR intervals are equal.
5. All other intervals and segments are within normal ranges.

6. Premature Atrial Contraction (PAC):

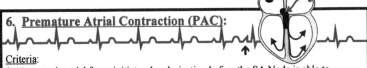

Criteria:
1. An ectopic atrial focus initiates depolarization before the SA Node is able to.
2. This causes a temporary shortening of the RR Interval.
NOTE: **The ectopic P'-wave shape is different from the SA Nodal P-wave shape**.

7. Wandering Pacemaker:

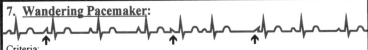

Criteria:
1. The SA Node is unable to initiate depolarizations
2. A series of ectopic atrial foci initiate depolarizations to compensate.
NOTE: **The ectopic P'-wave shapes are all different from each other**.
3. There is a regular rate (60-100bpm), but an irregular rhythm (unequal RR Intervals).

8. Multifocal Atrial Tachycardia (MAT):

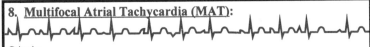

Criteria:
1. The SA Node is unable to initiate depolarizations.
2. A series of ectopic atrial foci initiate tachycardic depolarizations to compensate.
NOTE: **The ectopic P'-wave shapes are all different from each other**.
3. If all P-wave shapes are the same, but different from the SA Nodal P-wave shape,
    then it is called **"Unifocal Atrial Tachycardia,"** or just **"Atrial Tachycardia."**
4. The rate is tachycardic (>100bpm), with an irregular rhythm (unequal RR-Intervals).

9. Atrial Flutter (A-Flutter):

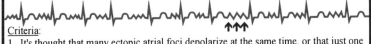

Criteria:
1. It's thought that many ectopic atrial foci depolarize at the same time, or that just one
    irritated ectopic atrial foci depolarizes continuously to cause multiple P'-waves.
NOTE: **Multiple P'-waves form a "Sawtooth" pattern; often called "F-waves."**
2. Depolarization conduction gets partially blocked at the entrance to the AV Node.
3. The atrial rate is tachycardic (250-400bpm), but the ventricular rate is much slower.
NOTE: **A-Flutter is described as a ratio of Atrial rate to Ventricular rate**.
    Common AV rate ratios are 2:1, 3:1, and 4:1; the ratio can be constant or can vary.
4. The rhythm is regular only if the AV rate ratio is constant, otherwise it is irregular.

10. Atrial Fibrillation (AF) (A-Fib):

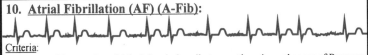

Criteria:
1. Innumerable ectopic atrial foci depolarize all at once; there is an absence of P-waves.
2. Depolarization conduction gets partially blocked at the entrance to the AV Node.
3. The atrial rate is fibrillating (>400bpm), but the ventricular rate is variable, it may be
    bradycardic, normal, or tachycardic.
4. If the rate is tachycardic, then the condition is called **"Rapid A-Fib,"** this is a life
    threatening situation and emergency treatment is necessary.
NOTE: **The Rhythm of A-Fib is traditionally described as Irregularly Irregular.**

B. Alternative Pathways of Atrial Depolarizations:

---

1. Wolff-Parkinson-White (WPW):
"Pre-Excitation"

Delta wave:

Anatomy: **Accessory conduction pathway** from any atria directly to any ventricle.
Physiology: **Antegrade** conduction of SA Nodal depolarizations from atria directly to ventricles via accessory pathway (bypassing the AV Node).
Criteria:
1. **Short PR Interval** (.<0.12s); P-wave may be inverted.
2. **Delta wave** present because both ventricles do not depolarized at the same moment.
3. **Wide QRS complex** (due to Delta wave).
NOTE:
If the accessory pathway conducts in a retrograde direction, and the AV Node conducts in an antegrade direction, then a tachycardia arrythmia similar to the Circus Movement Tachycardia (CMT) will result. This "Retrograde WPW" is a common cause of **PSVT**.

---

2. Circus Movement Tachycardia (CMT):
(Concealed Retrograde Bypass Circuit Tachycardia)

Anatomy: **Accessory conduction pathway(s)** from any atria directly to any ventricle.
Physiology: a **PAC** initiates atrial depolarizations which travel **Antegrade** through the AV Node to cause ventricular depolarizations. These depolarizations are then conducted **Retrograde** from the ventricles to the atria via the accessory pathway (bypassing the AV Node). This cycle repeats.
Criteria:
1. Rate **150-250**bpm.
2. **Normal PR Interval**; **Inverted P'-waves** in the ST segment of leads II,III,aVF.
3. **Narrow QRS complexes**; both ventricles depolarize at the same moment.
NOTE: Circus Movement Tachycardia is a very common cause of **PSVT**.

---

3. AV Nodal Reentry Tachycardia (AVNRT):

Anatomy: The **AV Node** is devided into two tracts: Slow (——) and Fast (- - -).
Physiology: a **PAC** initiates atrial depolarizations which travel via the slow AV Node path (the fast path is refractory due to previous SA Nodal depolarization). At the AV Node exit, depolarizations travel **Antegrade** to depolarize the ventricles, and **Retrograde** up the fast path to depolarize the atria. This cycle repeats.
Criteria:
1. Rate **100-300**bpm.
2. P'-wave hidden by QRS complex (atria and ventricles depolarize simultaneously).
3. P'-wave sometimes located at terminal portion of QRS complex (leads II, II, aVF).
NOTE: AV Nodal Reentry Tachycardia is the most common cause of **PSVT**.

C. AV Nodal (Junctional) Depolarizations:

1. Sinus Block with Ectopic Junctional Escape Beat: (see Conduction Block chapter)

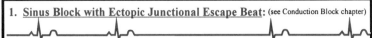

Criteria:
1. There is an abnormal pause after the T-wave due to lack of an SA Nodal P-wave, this causes a temporary lengthening of the RR Interval.
2. Since the SA Node refuses to initiate depolarization, and there are no atrial ectopic foci that initiate depolarizations, then the pause is broken by a new depolarization initiated by an AV Nodal ectopic focus. Normal sinus rhythm is then restored.
3. Narrow QRS complex.

2. Sinus Arrest with Junctional Escape Rhythm :

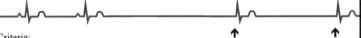

Criteria:
1. **Sinus arrest** (no P-wave) with no atrial ectopic foci contributing depolarizations.
2. **AV Nodal Ectopic focus** generates depolarizations at the **Idiojunctional rate**.
3. **Idiojunctional Rate = 40-60bpm**; rhythm is regular (all RR Intervals are equal).
4. **Narrow QRS complexes**.
5. T-waves are normal, except if there is retrograde conduction from AV Nodal ectopic focus, then atrial depolarization P'-wave will appear as a bump on the T-wave.

3. Premature Junctional Contraction (PJC):

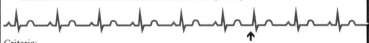

Criteria:
1. An AV Nodal ectopic focus initiates depolarization before the SA Node is able to.
2. There is no P-wave for this beat.
3. Normal QRS complex.
4. This causes a temporary shortening of the RR Interval.

4. Nonparoxysmal Junctional Tachycardia:

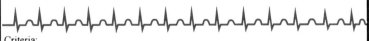

Criteria:
1. The SA Node is unable to initiate depolarizations.
2. No P-waves.
3. An Ectopic AV Nodal foci with enhanced automaticity generates depolarizations at a rate greater than the ideojunctional rate ("accelerated idiojunctional rate").
4. Rate is tachycardic **150-200bpm**, rhythm is regular (all RR Intervals are equal).
5. Narrow QRS complexes.
6. This rate and rhythm are sustained.

D. <u>Ventricular Depolarizations</u>:

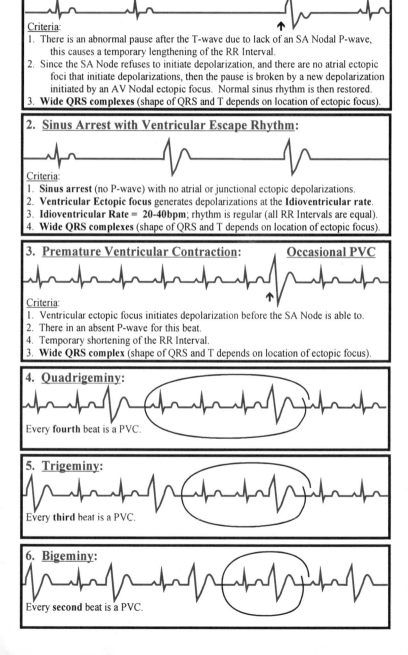

1. <u>Sinus Block with Ectopic Ventricular Escape Beat:</u> (see Conduction Block chapter)

<u>Criteria</u>:
1. There is an abnormal pause after the T-wave due to lack of an SA Nodal P-wave, this causes a temporary lengthening of the RR Interval.
2. Since the SA Node refuses to initiate depolarization, and there are no atrial ectopic foci that initiate depolarizations, then the pause is broken by a new depolarization initiated by an AV Nodal ectopic focus. Normal sinus rhythm is then restored.
3. **Wide QRS complexes** (shape of QRS and T depends on location of ectopic focus).

2. <u>Sinus Arrest with Ventricular Escape Rhythm</u>:

<u>Criteria</u>:
1. **Sinus arrest** (no P-wave) with no atrial or junctional ectopic depolarizations.
2. **Ventricular Ectopic focus** generates depolarizations at the **Idioventricular rate**.
3. **Idioventricular Rate = 20-40bpm**; rhythm is regular (all RR Intervals are equal).
4. **Wide QRS complexes** (shape of QRS and T depends on location of ectopic focus).

3. <u>Premature Ventricular Contraction</u>: <u>Occasional PVC</u>

<u>Criteria</u>:
1. Ventricular ectopic focus initiates depolarization before the SA Node is able to.
2. There in an absent P-wave for this beat.
4. Temporary shortening of the RR Interval.
3. **Wide QRS complex** (shape of QRS and T depends on location of ectopic focus).

4. <u>Quadrigeminy</u>:
Every **fourth** beat is a PVC.

5. <u>Trigeminy</u>:
Every **third** beat is a PVC.

6. <u>Bigeminy</u>:
Every **second** beat is a PVC.

7. <u>Run of PVC's</u>:

NOTE:
1. This is a transient run of ventricular tachycardia.
2. Less than 6 PVC's in a row is considered a "short run."
3. More than 6 PVC's in a row is considered pathological.

8. <u>Ventricular Tachycardia</u>:

<u>Criteria</u>:
1. May have pulse or no pulse.
2. Ventricular **Rate = 150-250 bpm**.
3. Wide QRS complexes, no P-waves.
4. RR intervals approximately equal.

Unifocal:
One ectopic focus: all QRS same shape.

Multifocal:
Two or more ectopic foci: repetition of corresponding QRS shapes.

<u>Unifocal (monomorphic):</u>
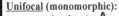

<u>Multifocal (polymorphic):</u>
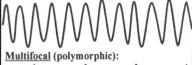

9. <u>Torsades de Pointes</u> Ventricular Tachycardia: "Twisting of the Points"

<u>Criteria</u>:
1. Wave form amplitude oscillates around isoelectric baseline.
2. Induced by extreme QT Interval prolongation.
3. Sometimes seen in: quinidine toxicity, hypomagnesemia, tricyclic overdose, etc.

10. <u>Ventricular Fibrillation</u>:

<u>Criteria</u>:
1. No Pulse.
2. Not able to determine EKG isoelectric baseline.
3. Low amplitude chaotic rapid EKG (ventricular rate >250bpm).

11. <u>Pulseless Electrical Activity</u> (PEA)
<u>Electro-Mechanical Dissociation</u> (EMD):

<u>Criteria</u>:
1. **No pulse** (the dying heart has remnant electrical activity, but no mechanical activity).
2. EKG shows a weak, low amplitude, slow rate signal with regular rhythm.
3. There is no characteristic wave form shape, but the shape is consistent in each lead.

12. <u>Asystole</u>: "Flat Line"

NOTE:
1. There is no electrical activity (no EKG signal), and no mechanical activity (no pulse).
2. Electrical shock therapy is ineffective to restore any EKG rhythm.
3. Medicine therapy may restore some EKG rhythm.

III. ARRHYTHMIAS ORGANIZED BY RATE:

A. Bradycardic Arrhythmias:

Atrial:
1. Sinus Bradycardia
2. Sinus Block with atrial escape beat
3. Sick Sinus Syndrome

Junctional:
4. Sinus Block with junctional escape beat
5. Sinus Arrest with junctional rhythm
6. AV Blocks

Ventricular:
7. Sinus Block with ventricular escape beat
8. Sinus Arrest with ventricular escape rhythm
9. PED and EMD
10. Asystole

B. Normocardic Arrhythmias:

Atrial:
1. Normal Sinus Rhythm (NSR)
2. Sinus Arrhythmia (physiologic)
3. Premature Atrial Contraction (PAC)
4. Wandering Pacemaker

Supraventricular:
5. Wolff-Parkinson-White (WPW) Pre-excitation

Junctional:
6. Premature Junctional Contraction (PJC)

Ventricular:
7. Occasional PVC
8. Quadrigeminy
9. Trigeminy
10. Bigeminy

C. Tachycardic Arryhthmias:

Atrial **Narrow** QRS complex Tachycardia:
1. Sinus Tachycardia [>100bpm]
2. Multifocal Atrial Tachycardia (MAT) [>100bpm]
3. Atrial Flutter [sometimes >100bpm]
4. Rapid Atrial Fibrillation (Rapid A-Fib or Rapid AF) [>100bpm]

Paroxysmal Supraventricular Tacycardia (PSVT) **Narrow** QRS Complex Tachycardia:
(Note: the term "Paroxysmal Atrial Tachycardia" (PAT) is no longer used)
5. Retrograde WPW [150-250bpm]
6. Circus Movement Tachycardia (CMT) [150-250bpm]
7. AV Node Reentry Tachycardia (AVNRT) [150-300bpm]

Junctional **Narrow** QRS Complex Tachycardia:
8. Non Paroxysmal Junctional Tachycardia (NPJT) [150-200bpm]

Ventricular **Wide** QRS complex Tachycardia:
9. Run of PVC's [>100bpm]
10. Ventricular Tachycardia (unifocal, multifocal) [150-250bpm]
11. Torsades de Pointes [150-250bpm]
12. Ventricular Fibrillation [>250bpm]

CHAPTER 7

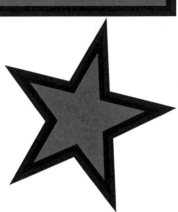

SPECIAL TOPICS:

SPECIAL TOPICS

44

I. ELECTROLYTE IMBALANCES:

hyperparathyroid

CALCIUM

HypoCalcemia ($\Downarrow$Ca++): Low Calcium
Criteria:
Prolonged QT Interval (**QT > 0.4sec**).
   (Late Repolarization)
Leads:
Most Precordial V1-V6

HyperCalcemia ($\Uparrow$Ca++): Low Calcium
Criteria:
Short QT Interval (approx **QT < 0.3sec**).
   (Early Repolarization)
Leads:
Most Precordial V1-V6

ACE, Lasix

POTASIUM

HypoKalemia ($\Downarrow$K+): Low Potassium
Criteria:
1. T-wave Flat (low amplitude) or Inverted.
2. U-wave (supplemental wave after T, before P)
Leads:
Most Precordial V1-V6

U-Wave

HyperKalemia ($\Uparrow$K+): High Potassium
Criteria:
T-waves are Tall ("Peaked" or "Tented")
Leads:
Most Precordial V1-V6

II. DRUG EFFECTS:

Digoxin:
Mechanism:
   Digoxin slows conduction at the AV-Node.
   HypoKalemia worsens Digoxin Toxicity.
Criteria:
   1. Bradycardia.
   2. ST Segment Depression with down slope.
   3. Toxicity: AV Block or Junctional Rhythm occur; Ventricular Tachycardia possible.
Leads:
   Best seen in Limb Lead I, and Precordial Leads V5, V6.

Quinidine:
Mechanism:
   Quinidine slows repolarization.
Criteria:
   1. P-waves wide, sometimes double-peaked.
   2. QRS Complex wide.
   3. QT Interval prolonged.
   4. T-waves flat, inverted, or with U-wave.
   5. Bradycardia.
   6. Toxicity: Complete AV Block may occur; Torsades de Pointes arrhythmia may occur.
Leads:
   Best seen in Limb Lead I, and Precordial Leads V5, V6.

III. HYPOTHERMIA:

Criteria:
1. **J-wave** ("Osborn wave") present at end of QRS.
   Also known as :J-Point Elevation."

Leads:
Limb Leads II, III, aVF
sometimes Precordial Leads also

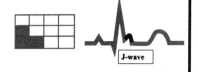

IV. PULMONARY EMBOLISM ("S1-Q3"):

Criteria:
1. **S-wave** Deep in Limb Lead I.
2. **ST Segment Depression** in Lead II.
3. **Q-wave** significant in Lead III.
4. **T-wave Inversion** in Lead III.

Leads:
Limb Leads I, II, III.

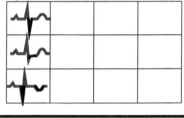

V. ARTIFACTS, ETC.:

1. **Standardization marks:** ⌐Full standard:10mm=1mV. ⌐⌐Full standard limb leads, half standard precordial leads.

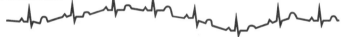

2. **Changing Baseline:** Poor electrode contact with patient's skin (hair, dirt, oils, not enough conduction gel, etc.).

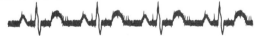

3. **Electrical Interference:** Some interfering electrical current at or near the patient's bedside.

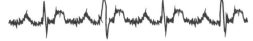

4. **Muscle Tremor, muscle movement:** Patient is tense, moving or trembling: EKG may show bizarre waveforms.

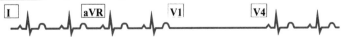

5. **Absent Leads:** Will give "Flat Line" appearance:

| I | aVR | V1 | V4 |

6. **Improper or reversed electrode placement:** EKG tracing may appear correct:
   Look for subtle clues such as False poor R-wave progression, or False Axis deviation, etc.
   With any abnormal EKG tracing, the electrode placement should be checked before making any diagnosis.

CHAPTER 8

HEART MURMURS

48

I. EXAMINATION OF THE HEART

A. THE FOUR BASIC PRINCIPALS OF EXAMINATION:
1. **Inspection**: Looking
2. **Auscultation**: Listening
3. **Percussion**: Tapping and listening (to detect solid or hollow)
4. **Palpation**: Tactile perception. (to detect PMI, thrill, or heave)

B. THE BASIC FINDINGS UPON EXAMINATION:
1. **Heart rate**: regular, tachycardic or bradycardic
2. **Rhythm**: regular, irregular, or irregularly irregular
3. **Presence and quality of S1 and S2**
4. **Presence of a gallop (S3 or S4), or other heart sound**
5. **Presence of a murmur:**
   -Patient's position:
      Supine, Left Lateral Decubitus, Sitting.
   -Location heard best:
      Apex (mitral), Base right (aortic), Base left (pulmonic), Left Lower Sternal Border (tricuspid).
   -Loudness:
      Scale of 1 to 6.
   -Stethoscope:
      Diaphragm or Bell.
   -Pitch:
      High, medium, low.
   -Quality:
      Harsh, blowing, rumbling, etc.
   -Radiation:
      To left axilla, to right neck, to apex, to right lower sternal border, etc.
   -Maneuvers which accentuate it or suppress it:
      Inspiration, expiration, valsalva, special position, squatting, standing, hand grasp.
6. **Location of the Point of Maximal Impulse {PMI}**: corresponds to apex:
   Normal PMI is located at 4th or 5th ICS in the mid-clavicular line {MCL}
7. **Presence of a Thrill, or a Heave:**
   Thrill is a vibration felt through bone (ribs, sternum); Heave is movement of chest wall.
8. **Presence of a Pericardial Friction Rub.**

C. **DETAILS OF THE EXAMINATION:**

1. **EXAMINATION STEP BY STEP BASED ON POSITION:**
   (A). **Examination in the Supine position:**
      (1). **Inspect:** for apex Point of Maximal Impulse {PMI}
         (normal PMI is located at 4th or 5th inter-costal space {ICS} in the mid-clavicular line {MCL}).
      (2). **Auscultate:** [use firm pressure on *Diaphragm* of stethoscope for high-pitched sounds]
         [use light pressure on *bell* of stethoscope for low-pitched sounds]
         <u>Aortic Area:</u> [2nd Right ICS at Right Sternal Border (at the right base of the heart)].
            Diaphragm will reveal:
               Aortic Regurgitation {AR}
               Aortic Stenosis {AS}.
         <u>Pulmonic Area:</u> [2nd Left ICS at Left Sternal Border (at the left base of the heart)].
            Diaphragm will reveal:
               Physiological S2 Splitting (A2 sound, P2 sound with inspiration)
               Pathological S2 Splitting (A2 sound, P2 sound heard with expiration)
               Pulmonic Regurgitation {PR}
               Pulmonic Stenosis {PS}
               Pericardial Friction Rub
               Patent Ductus Arteriosis {PDA}.
         <u>Tricuspid Area:</u> [Lower Left Sternal Border (or epigastrium/xiphoid area)].
            Diaphragm will reveal:
               S1 sound, S2 Sound
               Split S1 sound
               Tricuspid Regurgitation {TR}
               Tricuspid Stenosis {TS}.
            Bell will reveal:
               S3 Sound
               Tricuspid Stenosis {TS}.
         <u>Mitral Area:</u> [5th Left ICS at Mid-Clavicular Line (at the apex)].
            Diaphragm will reveal:
               S1 sound, S2 Sound
               Mitral Regurgitation {MR}
               Mitral Stenosis {Ms}
               Mid-Systolic Click From Mitral Prolapse
               Opening Snap {OS} of Mitral Stenosis {MS}
               Radiation of Aortic Regurgitation {AR}.
            Bell will reveal:
               S3 Sound
               S4 Sound
               Mitral Stenosis {MS}.
         <u>Auscultate for **Radiations**</u> if there is a murmur:
               To the **Right neck/carotid** for AS
               To the **Left neck** for PS
               To the **Left Axilla** for MR
               To the **Apex** for AR, and HSS.
               To the **Right sternal border** for TR, and **PR**
               To the **Left clavicle** for **PDA**
               To the **Back** for **Coarctation of the aorta**
   (3). **Percuss:**
      Determine size of the heart (this is rarely done).
   (4). **Palpate:**
      Fingertips for **Point of Maximal Impulse** {PMI}
         (normal PMI is located at 4th or 5th ICS in the mid-clavicular line {MCL})
      Palm placed on sternum for **Thrill**
         (vibrations of murmurs felt through bone)
      Heal of hand for **Heave**
         (abnormal elevations of chest wall due to abnormal contraction of the ventricles).

   (B). **Examination in the Left Lateral Decubitus Position:**
      (1). **Auscultate:**
         <u>Mitral Area:</u>
            Bell will most clearly reveal S3 Sound, S4 Sound, and Mitral Stenosis {MS}.

   (C). **Examination in the Sitting Up and Leaning Forward Position:**
      (1). **Auscultate:**
         <u>Aortic Area:</u>
            Diaphragm will reveal Aortic Stenosis {AS}.
         <u>Mitral Area:</u>
            Diaphragm will reveal the Radiation of Aortic Regurgitation {AR}.

HEART SOUNDS and GALLOPS:
(summary)

SYSTOLIC SOUNDS:

S1 SOUND
Closure of Mitral (M1) **and Tricuspid** (T1) valves at **beginning of Systole.**
SPLIT S1
(M1 then T1)

S2 SOUND
Closure of Aortic (A1) **and Pulmonic** (P1) valves at **beginning of Diastole.**
SPLIT S2
Physiologic Split S2
(A2 then P2)
Pathologic Split S2
-Heard in the presence of certain murmurs.
Wide Split S2 (A2 then P2)
Fixed Split S2 (A2 then P2)
Reversed Split S2 (P2 then A2), "Paradoxical Split S2"

DIASTOLIC SOUNDS:

PERICARDIAL KNOCK

S3 SOUND GALLOP
Physiologic S3:
Pathologic S3: "S3 Gallop," **"Ventricular Gallop,"** or "Protodiastolic Gallop"
-Heard in the presence of certain murmurs.
-Due to **ventricular overloading** from insufficient valves or CHF.

S4 SOUND GALLOP
Physiologic S4:
Pathologic S4: "S4 Gallop," or **"Atrial Gallop,"** or "Pre-systolic Gallop"
-Heard in the presence of certain murmurs.
-Due to **decreased ventricular compliance during atrial contraction.**
-**Never present in Atrial Fibrillation**: because there is no atrial contraction.

SUMMATION GALLOP

<u>HEART MURMURS:</u>
(summary)

<u>SYSTOLIC MURMURS</u>:

<u>MIDSYSTOLIC</u>
Aortic Stenosis {AS}
Midsystolic Click of **Mitral Valve Prolapse** {MVP}
         with late systolic murmur
Hypertrophic Subaortic Stenosis {HSS}
    a.k.a. Hypertrophic Cardiomyopathy {HCM}
    a.k.a. Idiopathic Hypertrophic Subaortic Stenosis {IHSS}
    a.k.a. Hypertrophic Obstructive Cardiomyopathy {HOCM}
    a.k.a. Muscular Subaortic Stenosis
Pulmonic Stenosis {PS}

<u>HOLOSYSTOLIC (PANSYSTOLIC)</u>
Mitral Regurgitation {MR} (insufficiency)
Tricuspid Regurgitation {TR} (insufficiency)
Ventricular Septal Defect {VSD}

<u>DIASTOLIC MURMURS</u>:

<u>EARLY DIASTOLIC DECRESCENDO</u>
Aortic Regurgitation {AR} (insufficiency)
Pulmonic Regurgitation {PR} (insufficiency)

<u>MID DIASTOLIC RUMBLING</u>
Mitral Stenosis {MS} with **Opening Snap** {OS}
Tricuspid Stenosis {TS}

<u>CONTINUOUS MURMURS</u>:
Pericardial Friction Rub
Patent Ductus Arteriosus
Coarctation of the Aorta

52

IV. DETAILS OF HEART SOUNDS:

A. SYSTOLIC SOUNDS:
1. S1 SOUND
NOTE: S1 sound corresponds to **closure of Mitral and Tricuspid valves at beginning of Systole**.
Best heard at: Mitral area (Apex)
Clinical: Normal
Increased by Mitral Stenosis {MS}, and by Tachycardia;
   Appears increased with the decreased S2 of AS.
Decreased by Mitral Regurgitation {MR}, by 1st degree heart block, and by CHF.
Irregularly Irregular S1 Rhythm and Sound is heard during Atrial Fibrillation {A Fib}
2. SPLIT S1 (M1 then T1)
NOTE: The Tricuspid valve (T1) sometimes lags slightly behind Mitral valve (M1) in its closure.
Best heard at: Tricuspid area (Left Lower Sternal Border); sometimes at apex.
Clinical: Insignificant
3. S2 SOUND
NOTE: S2 sound corresponds to **closure of Aortic and pulmonic valves at beginning of Diastole**.
Best heard at: Aortic or Pulmonic area (Base)
Clinical: Normal
Increased by none; but appears increased with the decreased S1 of MR.
Decreased by Aortic Stenosis {AS}; and appears decreased with the increased S1 of MS.
4. SPLIT S2
Physiologic Split S2 (A2 then P2)
NOTE: The Pulmonic valve (P2) sometimes lags slightly behind Aortic valve (A2) in its closure.
Best heard at: Pulmonic area (Left 2nd ICS).
Clinical: Insignificant
Increased by **inspiration** (inspiration always delays pulmonic closure)
Decreased by expiration (physiologic Split S2 disappears during expiration)
Pathologic Split S2 (heard in the presence of murmurs)
NOTE: When Pulmonic valve (P2) abnormally lags behind Aortic valve (A2) in its closure.
Best heard at: Pulmonic area (Left 2nd ICS).
Wide Split S2 (A2 then P2)
NOTE: This is a significant delay in closure of Pulmonic valve (P2).
Clinical: Occurs during **Pulmonic Stenosis** {PS}; or **RBBB**.
   Also occurs during Mitral regurgitation {MR} due to early Aortic valve (A2) closure.
Increased by **inspiration**
Decreased by expiration
Fixed Split (A2 then P2)
NOTE: This is a wide split S2 that **does not vary with respiration**.
Clinical: Occurs during **Atrial Septal Defect** {ASD}; or **Right Heart Failure**.
Increased by none
Decreased by none
Reversed Split (P2 then A2); "paradoxical Split S2"
NOTE: This occurs when **Aortic valve (A2) closes after the Pulmonic valve** (P2).
Clinical: Occurs during **LBBB**.
Increased by **Expiration**
Decreased by inspiration

B. DIASTOLIC SOUNDS:
1. PERICARDIAL KNOCK
NOTE: this is an Intra-cardiac sound similar to S4; but unlike the extra-cardiac pericardial friction rub.
Best heard at: Mitral area (apex).
Pitch = low
Bell is best
Quality = intense
Maneuvers
   -Position: patient in left lateral decubitus, use bell at apex to increase S3 sound.
   -Inspiration: Increases Knock sound.
Other
   -Early diastolic, follows S2.
   -Due to **constrictive pericarditis** causing **abrupt end to ventricular filling**.
   -Similar mechanism as S4 sound, but knock may occur with Atrial Fibrillation.

2. S3 SOUND

Physiologic S3:

Best heard at: Mitral area (apex).

Pitch = low

Bell is best

Quality := dull

Maneuvers

-Position: patient in left lateral decubitus, use bell at apex to increase S3 sound.

Other

-Early diastole, follows S2.

-Common in children.

-Common in 3rd trimester pregnancy.

Pathologic S3: "S3 Gallop" or **"Ventricular Gallop"** (heard in the presence of murmurs)

Best heard at: Mitral area (apex).

Pitch = low

Bell is best

Quality := dull

Maneuvers

-Positions:

Left S3: patient in left lateral decubitus, exhaling, use bell at apex to increase S3.

Right S3: patient supine, inhaling, best heard at left lower sternal border.

-Inspiration: Increases Right S3 sound.

-Expiration: Increases Left S3 sound.

Other

-Early diastole, follows S2

-Patient is usually over 40 years old.

-Common in **MR** or **TR** or **heart failure** due to **ventricular overloading**.

3. S4 SOUND

Physiologic S4:

Best heard at: Mitral area (apex).

Pitch = low

Bell is best

Quality := dull

Maneuvers

-Positions: patient in left lateral decubitus, use bell at apex to increase S4.

-Expiration: Increases S4 sound.

Other

-Late diastole, precedes S1.

-Due to **ventricular hypertrophy during atrial contraction**.

-Common in **athletes**.

Pathologic S4: "S4 Gallop," **"Atrial Gallop"** or "Pre-systolic Gallop" (heard in the presence of murmurs)

Best heard at: Mitral area (apex).

Pitch = low

Bell is best

Quality := dull

Maneuvers

-Positions:

Left S4: patient in left lateral decubitus, exhaling, use bell at apex to increase S4.

Right S4: patient supine, inhaling, best heard at left lower sternal border.

-Expiration: Increases Left S4 sound.

-Inhalation: Increases Right S4 sound

Other

-Late diastole, precedes S1.

-*Large A-wave* in jugular veins.

-Due to **decreased ventricular compliance during atrial contraction**

-Common in:

AS

HSS

Severe Hypertension

Coronary Artery Disease {CAD} leading to **Ischemia** or **MI**

-**Never present in Atrial Fibrillation**: because there is no atrial contraction.

4. SUMMATION GALLOP

-Quadruple Rhythm occurs when both S3 and S4 are present with S1 and S2.

-During rapid heart rates, S3 and S4 may blend together as a"Summation."

-Never present during Atrial Fibrillation: because there is no atrial contraction, no S4.

V. DETAILS OF HEART MURMURS:

A. SYSTOLIC MURMURS:

1. EJECTION MURMURS

   Ejection murmurs are associated with blood turbulence or obstruction while the blood is leaving the heart. These murmurs are usually associated with radiations, and always associated with systole.

   Systolic ejection murmurs
   - Aortic Stenosis {AS}
   - Hypertrophic Sub-aortic Stenosis {HSS}
   - Pulmonic Stenosis {PS}

2. MIDSYSTOLIC

   Aortic Stenosis {AS}

   Best heard at: Aortic area (Base)

   Pitch = medium

   Diaphragm is best

   Radiation: to Right neck/carotid, sometimes to left sternal border

   Quality = Harsh

   Maneuvers
   - -Palpation: Loud AS murmur will have a thrill.
   - -Position: patient sitting and leaning forward to increase AS murmur.
   - -Expiration: Increases murmur.
   - -Amyl Nitrite inhalation: Increases murmur.

   Other
   - -S2 sound is decreased
   - -S4 sound at apex is common

   Midsystolic Click of **Mitral Valve Prolapse** {MVP} with late systolic murmur

   NOTE: Click is not always associated with a murmur.

   When murmur is present:
   - -Indicates mitral regurgitation.
   - -Is indication for antibiotic prophylaxis during certain situations (e.g. dental work).

   Best heard at: Mitral area (Apex)

   Pitch = High pitched "click" sound.

   Diaphragm is best

   Maneuvers:
   - -Squatting: will delay the click/murmur.
   - -Standing: will make the click/murmur early systolic.
   - -Valsalva: Increases the click/murmur.

   Hypertrophic Subaortic Stenosis {HSS}

   aka Hypertrophic Cardiomyopathy {HCM}

   aka Idiopathic Hypertrophic Subaortic Stenosis {IHSS}

   aka Hypertrophic Obstructive Cardiomyopathy {HOCM}

   aka Muscular Subaortic Stenosis

   Best heard at: Left Sternal Border (3rd to 4th ICS)

   Pitch = medium

   Diaphragm is best

   Radiation: to Apex

   Quality = Harsh

   Maneuvers
   - -Squatting: Decreases murmur.
   - -Standing: Increases murmur.
   - -Valsalva: Increases murmur.
   - -Handgrips: Decreases murmur.

   Other
   - -S4 sound at apex is common.

   Pulmonic Stenosis {PS}

   NOTE: very rare.

   Best heard at: Pulmonic area (Base)

   Pitch = Medium

   Diaphragm is best

   Radiation: to left neck

   Quality = Harsh

   Maneuvers
   - -Palpation: Loud PS murmur will have a thrill.
   - -Inspiration: Increases murmur.

3. HOLOSYSTOLIC (PANSYSTOLIC)

Mitral Regurgitation {MR} (insufficiency)
- <u>Best heard at</u>: Mitral area (apex)
- <u>Pitch</u> = medium
- <u>Diaphragm</u> is best
- <u>Radiation</u>: to Left axilla.
- <u>Quality</u> =.Blowing
- <u>Maneuvers</u>
  - -Expiration: Increases murmur.
  - -Amyl Nitrite inhalation: Decreases murmur.
- <u>Other</u>
  - -S1 sound is decreased
  - -S3 sound at apex is common (Ventricular overload)

Tricuspid Regurgitation {TR} (insufficiency)
- <u>Best heard at</u>: Tricuspid area
- <u>Pitch</u> = medium
- <u>Diaphragm</u> is best
- <u>Radiation</u>: to Right sternal border or Right mid-clavicular line
- <u>Quality</u> = Blowing
- <u>Maneuvers</u>
  - -Inspiration: Increases murmur
- <u>Other</u>
  - -S3 sound at tricuspid area is common
  - **-Large *V*-wave** in Jugular Veins

Ventricular Septal Defect {VSD}
- <u>Best heard at</u>: along left sternal border (3rd-4th ICS)
- <u>Pitch</u> = High
- <u>Diaphragm</u> is best
- <u>Radiation</u>: variable
- <u>Quality</u> = Harsh
- <u>Maneuvers</u>
  - -Palpation: Loud VSD murmur will have a thrill.
  - -Amyl Nitrite inhalation: Decreases murmur.
- <u>Other</u>
  - -Occurs mostly in young children.
  - -May be a component of Tetralogy of Fallot.
  - **-Eisenmenger Syndrome**:
    - ASD or VSD or PDA with obstructive pulmonary HTN, cyanosis, right to left shunt.

B. DIASTOLIC:

1. EARLY DIASTOLIC DECRESCENDO:

Aortic Regurgitation {AR} (insufficiency)
- <u>Best heard at</u>: Aortic area (Base)
- <u>Pitch</u> = High
- <u>Diaphragm</u> is best
- <u>Radiation</u>: to Apex
- <u>Quality</u>: = Blowing
- <u>Maneuvers</u>
  - -Position: patient sitting and leaning forward, exhales to increase AR murmur.
  - -Expiration: Increases murmur.
  - -Amyl Nitrite inhalation: Decreases murmur.
- <u>Other</u>
  - **-S3 or S4 sound** at apex during severe regurgitation
  - -PMI may be displaced inferiolaterally, or widened in diameter.
  - -Widened pulse pressure: Large and bounding pulse, **"Water-Hammer Pulse"**
  - **-Austin Flint Murmur** = regurgitant flow banging against mitral valve.
  - **-Midsystolic Murmur** = volume overloaded left ventricle ejects excess blood.
  - **-Duroziez Murmur** = a double murmur over the femoral artery due to AR.

Pulmonic Regurgitation {PR} (insufficiency)
- <u>NOTE</u>: rare, and usually of no clinical consequence.
- <u>Best heard at</u>: Pulmonic area (Base)
- <u>Pitch</u> = High
- <u>Diaphragm</u> is best
- <u>Radiation</u>: to Right lower sternal border
- <u>Quality</u>: = Blowing
- <u>Maneuvers</u>
  - -Inspiration: Increases murmur
- <u>Other</u>
  - **-Graham Steell Murmur**: when PR is due to Pulmonary hypertension:
    - (Early Diastolic Decrescendo along left sternal border).

3. MID DIASTOLIC RUMBLING

Mitral Stenosis {MS} with Opening Snap {OS}

Best heard at: Mitral Area (Apex)

Pitch = Low (but OS is high pitched "snap" sound)

Bell is best

Radiation: none

Quality = Rumbling

Maneuvers

-Position: patient in left lateral decubitus, use bell at apex to increase MS murmur.

-Exhalation: Increases murmur.

Other

-**S1 is characteristically loud,** especially at the apex.

-S2 often absent.

-**Opening Snap** {OS}: follows S2 and initiates the murmur (occurs when stiff mitral valve opens).

Tricuspid Stenosis {TS} NOTE: Tricuspid stenosis is uncommon; usually associated with mitral stenosis.

Best heard at: Tricuspid Area

Pitch = Low

Bell is best

Radiation: none

Quality = Rumbling

Maneuvers

-Inspiration: Increases murmur.

-Exhalation: Decreases murmur.

-Valsalva: Decreases murmur.

Other

-**Large *A-waves*** in jugular veins.

-JVD

-Opening Snap {OS}: may be present but is difficult to assess in TS

-Carvallo's Sign: inspiration while sitting upright to accentuate TS murmur.

C. CONTINUOUS MURMURS:

Pericardial Friction Rub NOTE: this is an "Extra-cardiac" Sound, due to pericardial inflammation.

Best heard at: Pulmonic area

Pitch = High

Diaphragm is best

Radiation: none

Quality: = Scratching

Maneuvers

-Position: patient sitting up and leaning forward to increase Rub.

-Inhalation: Increases Rub.

Patent Ductus Arteriosus

Best heard at: Pulmonic area in late systole

Pitch = medium

Diaphragm is best

Radiation: to Left clavicle

Quality: = Harsh: **"Machinery"** sound

Maneuvers

-Palpation: Loud PDA murmur will have a thrill.

-Valsalva: Increases murmur.

-Amyl Nitrite inhalation: Decreases murmur.

Other

-S2 may be obscured by the murmur.

-Widened pulse pressure: Large and bounding pulse, **"Water-Hammer Pulse"**

-**Machinery Murmur** = cliche for the murmur of PDA.

-**Eisenmenger Syndrome**:

ASD or VSD or PDA with obstructive pulmonary HTN, cyanosis, right to left shunt.

-**Systolic Murmur** without Diastalic component occurs with pulmonary HTN.

Coarctation of the Aorta

Best heard at: Pulmonic Area

Pitch = medium

Diaphragm is best

Radiation: to Back along Left Thoracic Spinous Processes.

Quality:= Harsh

Maneuvers

-Palpation: Loud Coarctation murmur will have a thrill.

Other

-Systolic Murmur without diastolic component indicates less stenosis.

-Continuous Murmur on Lateral Chest wall indicates significant pressure and dilated collateral vessels.

-**"3 Sign"** X-ray shows pre- and post-stenotic dilatation of Aorta.

-**Rib-Notching**: X-ray shows notched ribs due to dilated collateral vessels.

-Absent femoral pulses.

-Elevated BP in upper extremities is common.

ABBREVIATIONS

A1 Aortic valve opening
A2 Aortic valve closure
AF Atrial Fibrillation
A-Fib Atrial Fibrillation
A-Flutter Atrial Flutter
AR Aortic regurgitation
AS Aortic stenosis
ASD Atrial septal defect
AV Atrial-ventricular
AVNRT AV Nodal reentrant tachycardia
BBB Bundle branch block
bpm beats per minute
CMT Circus movement tachycardia
ECG Electrocardiogram
EKG Electrocardiogram
EMD Electro-mechanical dissociation
HCM Hypertrophic cardiomyopathy
HCOM Hypertrophic obstructive cardiomyopathy
HSS Hypertrophic subaortic stenosis
HTN Hypertension
ICS Intercostal space
IHSS Idiopathic Hypertrophic subaortic stenosis
JVD Jugular venous distention
LAH Left anterior hemiblock
LBBB Left bundle branch block
LPH Left posterior hemiblock
M1 Mitral valve closure
MR Mitral regurgitation
MS Mitral stenosis
Mv Millivolts
MVP Mitral valve prolapse
NSR Normal sinus rhythm
OS Opening snap
P1 Pulmonic valve opening
P2 Pulmonic valve closure
PAC Premature atrial contraction
PDA Patent Ductus Arteriosus
PEA Pulseless electrical activity
PJC Premature junctional contraction
PMI Point of maximal impulse
PR Pulmonic regurgitation
PS Pulmonic stenosis
PSVT Paroxysmal supraventricular tachycardia
PVC Premature ventricular contraction
RBBB Right bundle branch block
s seconds
SA Sino-atrial
T1 Tricuspid valve closure
TR Tricuspid regurgitation
TS Tricuspid stenosis
VSD Ventricular-septal defect
V-Fib Ventricular Fibrillation
WPW Wolff-Parkinson-White syndrome